GROUNDED

Discovering the missing piece
in the puzzle of children's behaviour

Claire Wilson

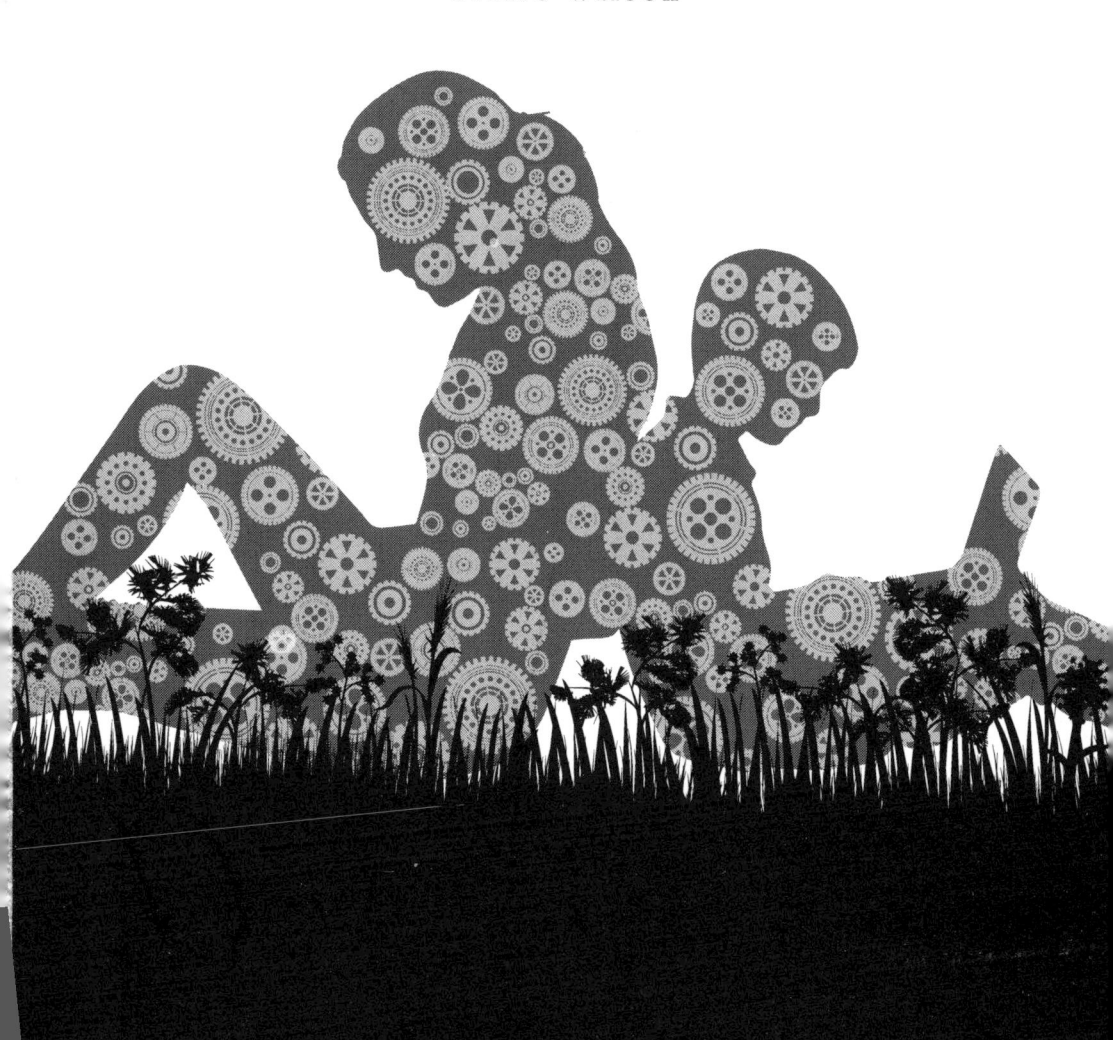

ISBN : 978-1-9164133-0-6
EISBN : 978-1-9164133-1-3
© 2018 Claire Wilson
All rights reserved

No portion of this book may be reproduced or transmitted in any form or by any means, electronic or mechanical, including photocopying, recording or by any information and storage retrieval system, except for brief quotations in reviews or articles, without the prior written permission of the copyright holder.

Note
The stories included in these pages are all based on real moments. Names and some other key details have been purposely changed to protect the identities and privacy of those discussed, but they are all from real people and real experiences. Real lives, living real life. I honour each person who has shared these moments with me over the years and given me permission to share their stories here.

Complete book design by Steve O'Brien
steve@1512design.com www.1512design.com
mobile: 07544 544195, tel: 0115 931 307

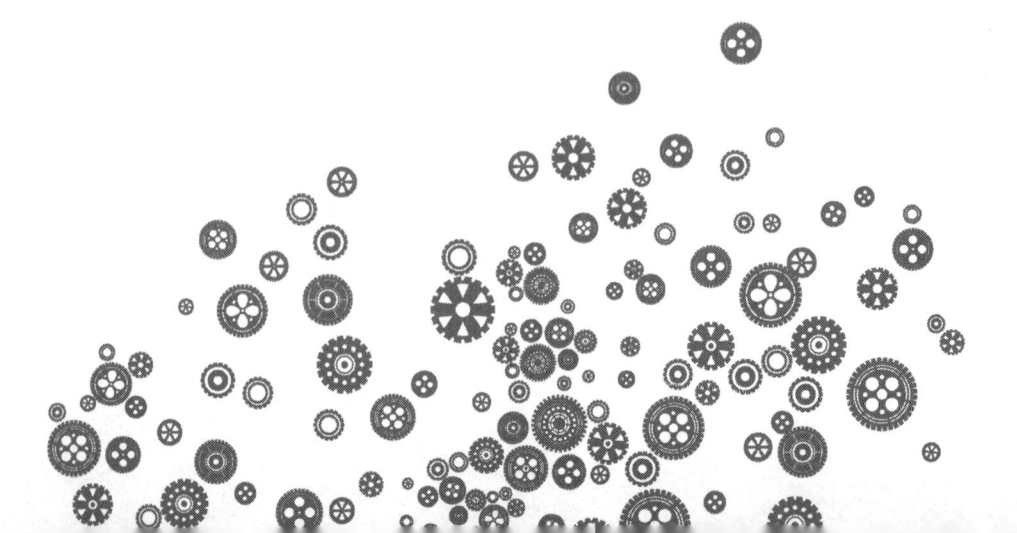

About Claire Wilson

"Claire Wilson is a passionate advocate for children. Through her trauma-informed approaches and unique insight, she always strives to understand the reasons behind a child's behaviour and what they are experiencing in both mind and body. With her expert guidance, my staff have been helped to identify ways to support our children and create a safe environment in which they can begin to thrive. My school is such a different place because of Claire and the support of CHEW Initiatives over the last few years."
Ruth Tonkinson, *Head Teacher*

"I felt like a huge weight had been lifted and the path forward looked a little clearer following our consultation with Claire. Our journey will have some twists and turns, I am sure, but having Claire in our corner helps immensely."
Dermot Doyle, *parent*

"If someone were to ask my opinion on the impact and importance of our sessions, then I would have to tell them they were HUGELY important and I wish that more parents were able to benefit as I have. Every school should have access to a professional like Claire and I have no doubt that families would be more connected and young people would have better mental well-being."
Sarah Collier, *parent*

"After working with Claire over a number of years, it is clear how fully committed she is to giving pupils a voice: whether she is working with their teachers, parents or whole class, children's best interests are at the centre of all she does. Her depth of knowledge and understanding of children has been instrumental in supporting staff to create the best learning environments possible in which their class can feel safe and thrive."

Sarah Yates, *Deputy Head*

"I have known and worked with Claire for over a decade. I have witnessed her deep care for her young clients and the parents and professionals she works with. In the introduction to this book, Claire writes 'I believe that no situation is too hard to navigate; no riddle too hard to solve; no language too foreign to learn; and no puzzle too hard to complete, when you have all the pieces.' I can vouch that these are more than just words; they are an honest expression of how Claire sees her work with children and families. I have witnessed her tenacity in persevering for the sake of her clients, and believe it is absolutely her core strength as a professional."

Dr Lynne Souter-Anderson
Fellow of NCS, BACP Senior Accredited Therapist, PTUK Senior Supervisor, AST Consultant Sandplay Therapist
Director, Bridging Creative Therapies Consultancy

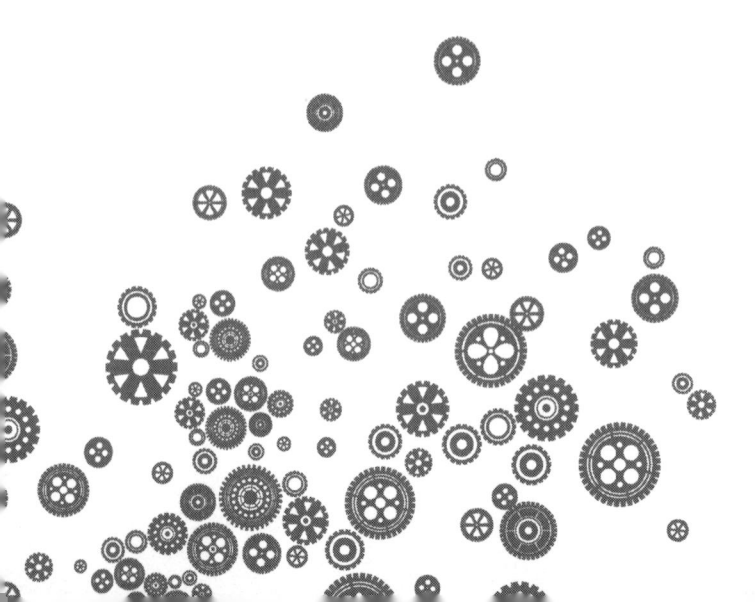

Contents

Introduction A Message For You		7

Section 1   What's really going on?

1	Lisa: A Lesson For Us All	11
2	The Common Answer	13
3	Help Is At Hand	15
4	The Big Question	17
5	Learning From The Animals	20
6	Getting Perspective	23
7	Neuroception In The Movies	32
8	It's Not Just The Children	38

Section 2   Understanding survival

9	F's For Survival	41
10	Social Engagement System	42
11	Mobilisation/Defence	47
12	Immobilisation – Shut-down – Freeze	54
13	Taking It All In	59
14	Can't Decide! (Functional Freeze)	60
15	Hearing	62
16	It Is Not A Conscious Choice	66
17	Don't Waste Your Time	70

Section 3   Grounded

18	Surviving When You Need To Survive	76
19	What Is Grounded?	78

20	What Stops Us Being The Calm, Grounded Adults We Want To Be?	81
21	What Helps Us Get Grounded?	87
22	Getting Grounded, Wrapping Presents	94
23	What's In A Smile?	97
24	Changing The Landscape	101

Section 4 Hope

25	The Benefits Of Grounded Adults	109
26	Supporting Narnia's Children	113
27	What Children Want	116
28	Jane's Special Story	118
29	Time For Timeout	120
30	From Me To You: A Message To All Who Read This	123
31	Revisiting Lisa	125
	References	127
	Additional Resources	130
	Partnership Programme	133

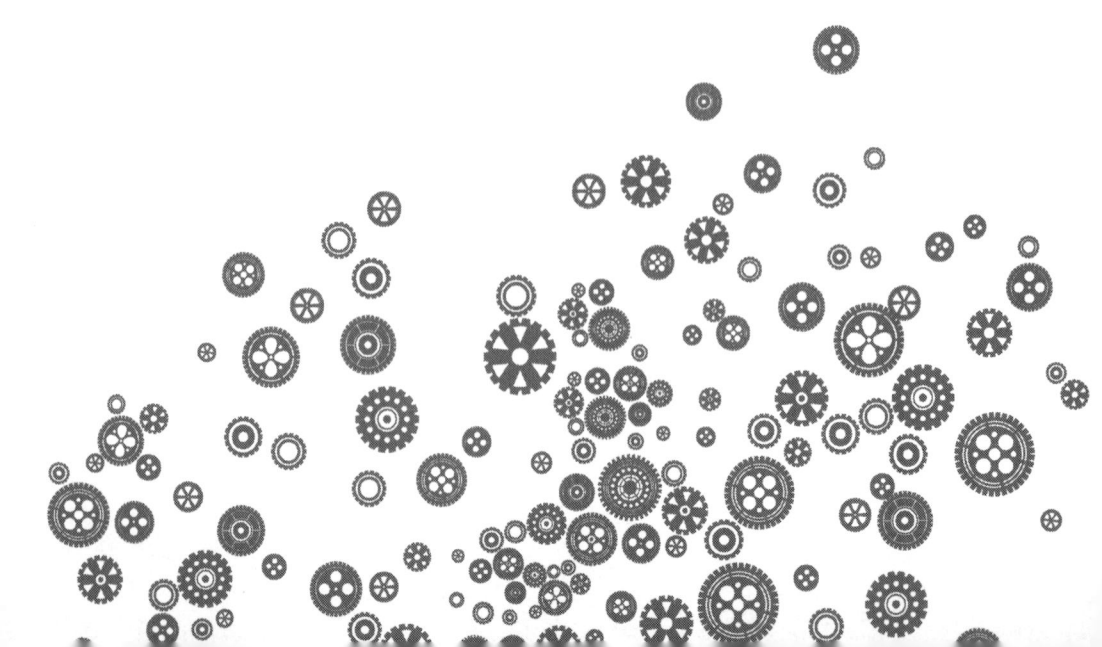

INTRODUCTION

A Message For You

If you are a parent, a professional who works with children, or someone who has children in your life who you care deeply about, then you are in the right place.

If you are one of the grown-ups who really want to know how to bring the best out of the children you are around, then you are not alone. Consider yourself among the huge movement of people worldwide who are prepared to learn and to grow themselves for the sake of the children precious to them.

If you feel you have come to a challenge, you don't understand what's going on with a child you know, and can't seem to get things to move forward no matter what you say or do – then I'm glad you are here. I wrote this book for you.

I believe that no situation is too hard to navigate; no riddle too hard to solve; no language too foreign to learn; and no puzzle too hard to complete, when you have all the pieces. And that's the thing. It may be that you have been putting your time and effort into completing your 'puzzle' with some crucial pieces missing. The old saying is often true: 'we don't know what we don't know'. It may just be that, up until now, you haven't explored things from this crucial perspective.

It started as a common thread in so many of the conversations I have had with parents and education and therapeutic professionals throughout my career so far. Whether we have been sat together in a classroom, staff room, quiet room or any of the various offices I have inhabited, as we explore what's going on with the child it is always something we speak about.

Initially, it was just an intuitive hunch that I offered as a possibility to be considered. However, my hunch sneaked its way into my Master's degree research and was powerfully verified. So, from that point on I have shared it, and the indisputable neuroscience behind it, as a fundamental piece of the puzzle. When we want to get better at understanding children, and especially how they behave when they are with us, then we need to understand, at a deeper level, who we are and what our very body is communicating to them.

My hope is that the words and stories I am going to share with you will encourage you on your journey. Even more than that, I hope they give you insight, understanding and practical ways forward so you can get back to moving ahead with the mission you have: to be a truly significant adult (for all the right reasons) in that child's life.

Is now a Good Time?
Before we really get going on this journey, I want to ask you, in all honesty: is now a good time?

Is now a good time for you to start to dig into these pages and these stories with me?

How are you doing?
Are you hungry? Thirsty? Tired? Done in?
I know that some conversations are best had at the right time. As the old wisdom says: 'there is a time for everything, and a season for every activity under the sun …' I don't know about you, but it's generally not a great idea to talk to me about anything important when I am overtired or hungry or in the middle of thinking deeply about something else. There *is* a good time for everything – and you get to decide if now is it for you.

I don't know what is going on for you in life at the moment, but if you feel overwhelmed, or if it is late and you are at the end of a really tough day, then maybe the best way to *look after you* right now is to go to sleep. The message in this book is *important* – but these words will keep until you are rested or fed, and ready for them.

Dealing with monkeys
I know that most of the parents and professionals with whom I have had the privilege to connect over the years are absolutely doing their best. I bet you are, too … and yet, if you are anything like most of them, I need to mention the monkey that may be lurking on your shoulder. Do you know the one? The monkey poised ready to whisper the 'not good enough' messages and swirl you up in a debilitating cloud of guilt for not being perfect?

The intention of these words is to help you. My hope is that they give you clarity and give you power. I am for your children, and I am for you! Please, if you know him, get that monkey on a short lead and don't let him twist any of the words in this book the wrong way.

Let's do it together
If you would like to hear me cheering you on as you get into these pages, then I'd love to serve you in that way. Please join the other parents and child-focused professionals (and people who are both) who have already signed up to be part of the *Grounded* book community. I can't wait to travel with you and share some honest and real stories from others who have journeyed through these pages. It's easy to join us: visit **www.groundedgrownups.com**.

Whether now is the time to read on or not, I am cheering for you. If now *is* a good time – you are awake, armed with a good cuppa, and ready for a chat – then let's get going. Let me tell you about Lisa.

SECTION 1

WHAT'S REALLY GOING ON?

One hundred years from now
It won't matter
What kind of car I drove
What kind of house I lived in
How much money I had in the bank
Nor what my clothes looked like
BUT
The world may be a little better
Because, I was important
In the life of a child.

From 'Within My Power' by Forest Witcraft

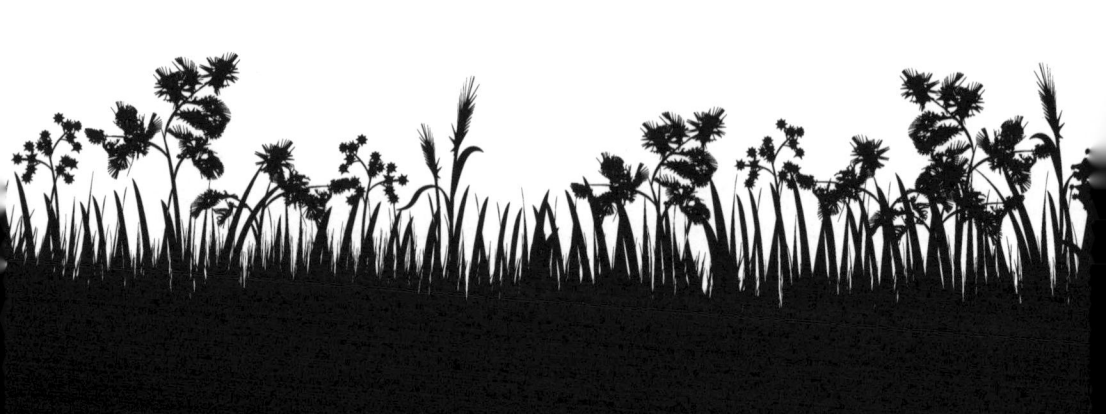

1

Lisa: A Lesson For Us All

They called her 'witch mummy'. But what hurt the most was that all three of her young daughters – her treasures, her world – would seek out her partner instead of her. *He* would be the one they would go to for a bedtime story. They fought over who would get to sit beside *him* to watch TV. *He* was the one they would talk to about their day at school, and *he* was the one they wanted to give them a goodnight kiss.

What doesn't kill you makes you stronger, they say. Well, she had been through hell. She had fought her own personal world war. She had set herself the mission of surviving three years of the most hideous onslaught from a neighbour – and she would keep her girls safe from him, too. It hadn't killed her – almost, when the firebomb came through the letter box, but not quite. And it hadn't made her stronger.

Sitting in a meeting – with her whole body shaking, staring at the floor, barely able to make an audible noise when she wanted to say something, her nail-bitten, trembling hands mindlessly obliterating a tissue – here she was, confessing her girls didn't listen to her, didn't like her and didn't want to be near her.

How was this right? How was it fair? She had given everything she had to get her little family through those years on her own. She lived to protect. She timed each leaving the flat to make sure he was out. She heard him cough through the wall and would gather the girls into the back room and play no-noise games. She stopped breathing. For three years she had held her breath and survived. She had mothered. She had sacrificed. She had protected.

Now there was no more threat. They were safe. Now he was gone. But so, too, were her relationships ... and that, that was killing her.

Not the norm, but just like us ...
Thankfully, what this precious mother went through is *not* the norm for billions who are parenting across the world today. Yes, there are those living in areas or circumstances where every day is a battle to survive, and there are many also living in relative safety. Whoever and wherever we are and whatever our circumstances, there is a profound lesson hidden within Lisa's story for us all – those who parent, those who teach and those who work with children in any other capacity.

If we take the time to explore and fathom what was happening with Lisa and her girls in those months after their neighbour's arrest, we will understand something that has the potential to make us all more effective in what we do with children.

Lisa's story didn't end there. But at this point, having given everything she possibly could to do her best for her children, she didn't know how to get her precious relationships restored. She knew her two older girls were struggling with things at school; reading was hard for one, and friendship issues were a constant challenge for the other. She desperately wanted to help them. They refused her. They wouldn't let her help them. They wouldn't come near.

If we can keep ourselves from judging her story on the few details we know, and if we instead honour this mum – whose full story we will never be able to fathom, who did what she could – then we will be able to embrace the wisdom she discovered, which is the message of this book, and apply it ourselves. However dramatic or however mundane our situations may be, we will understand how to bring out the best in the young ones around us ... and it will be with ease.

What Lisa discovered is something that is much more significant than any parenting gimmick, approach or strategy. It is beyond the latest technique or skills for 'behaviour management' in a classroom. This truth that we are going to explore together holds within it the potential for us to become who we really want to be: adults who make a positive, significant impact in the lives of the children we are around.

2

The Common Answer

Recently I was invited to sit on a panel as the Head, Deputy Head and Chair of Governors of a large primary school interviewed new teachers. I arrived with a head full of memories of all the times I'd been on the other side of the table. I felt honoured that now I was getting to do more than just sit, observe and give feedback: I was able to participate fully in asking questions. I had a blast! I love meeting people, connecting with them and helping bring out their best. I love asking good questions and I love going beneath the surface and finding out what makes each one of us unique.

Here's what is interesting: one of the questions the Head Teacher asked the candidates was: "If someone spent ten minutes in your classroom, what would you want them to know about you?"

It's a good question, eh?
So, let's play …

If I was to ask you the same question — whether for your classroom, your family home, your office or consulting room, or wherever else you connect with children — what would be your answer?

Don't turn the page until you have thought about your answer…

The answers the interview candidates gave to that question were, not surprisingly, as varied as their personalities. However, there was something that each and every candidate said:

'I'd want them to know I am approachable.'

This response was not something that made candidates stand out. It was not something that highlighted their uniqueness. On the contrary, it was a common desire, and I noticed it. It echoed the hearts of so many of the teachers I have worked with. It reminded me of my peers during my years of therapeutic training. And it reminded me of so many of the parents I've met around the world:

- The house mother in a children's home in Morocco who longed for her 'daughter' to talk to her about her nightmares.
- The now sole-custody dad who frequently told his boys 'whatever you are going through, you can always tell me'.
- The respectable, affluent mum of a teenage boy, longing for him to want to tell her about how hard he was finding life at that time.
- The small team of devoted locals spending their evenings in the same spot in an empty car park in the centre of a Brazilian town, waiting with water, medical supplies and huge pans of rice and stew until the street kids came out from their cardboard dens so they could help them.

Approachable. We want children to know they can come to us when things are hard. We want them to feel they have support in us. We want them to feel OK about moving towards us. We want to be approachable. If we parent or care for children in any way, we don't want children to have to 'go it alone'. We want to help them navigate the twists and turns of life, and for that we want them to come to us. We want to be a positive resource for them. We want to help them. We want to be in a relationship.

This is where – irrespective of language, culture, affluence or demographics – if we care about our children, we all have something in common. It is what we have in common with Lisa.

3

Help Is At Hand

Anyone who has been a parent knows what an unbelievably tough job it can be. Anyone who hasn't but works with parents or children can catch but a whiff of how physically, emotionally, mentally and spiritually hard parenting actually is at times. As is often said, it is the one job that carries such incredible responsibility and holds the potential to impact future generations, and yet for which there is no qualification or compulsory training.

Anyone who is a teacher or works with children in any role within an education establishment knows what a tough job it can be. Anyone who has never dealt with the dynamics of being responsible for 30+ bodies and brains in a confined space for six or seven hours a day can only imagine it (and they may, in all fairness, not want to!). There is no training that prepares you for the potential depletion of mental, physical and emotional resources as you work to support the little people, their parents, other professionals and *then* meet the work criteria under the perpetual threat of standards, achievement, progress and inspection.

Dreams mean work

Parents and professionals share a desire – a dream – to help our children feel supported and find ways to flourish, whatever life throws at them. The honest truth is that, whatever our role in the lives of children, it is not all glorious days, cuddles, high-fives, smiles or progress certificates. It can be hard. For those of us who really care about the children for whom we have responsibility, our role comes with the pressure of doing the best job we can – not because we should, or need to, but because we want to. Because we care. I know that sometimes it can feel like you are going it alone – or that the very system you are working in seems more about numbers than real lives with real stories.

I want to remind you that you are not on your own, and *there are people willing and able to support you.* Even the scientists in their ivory towers have help for us! Did you know that relatively recently there has been a significant breakthrough in the scientific understanding of neuroscience, neurophysiology and the neurophysiology of relationships?

No? Why? And what does all that mean in English? Well, whether or not we are parents, teachers or other child-focused professionals, if we want to understand more about being the approachable adults we want to be for children, we don't have to grope about in the dark, figuring out how to do it. If we want to be a positive influence for them, really helping to bring out their best, we don't have to 'wing it'. We don't have to hope for the best and we don't have to succumb to repeating generational patterns. The recent scientific breakthroughs can really help guide us. One of these has come from an incredible guy called Stephen Porges.

4

The Big Question

Dr Stephen Porges is a scientist and a worldwide-respected researcher who focuses his work in the fields of psychiatry and human development. He has shown us that children are obsessed with one question. One thing they are constantly working on. One program that is running on their metaphorical desktop all the time. Want to guess what it is?

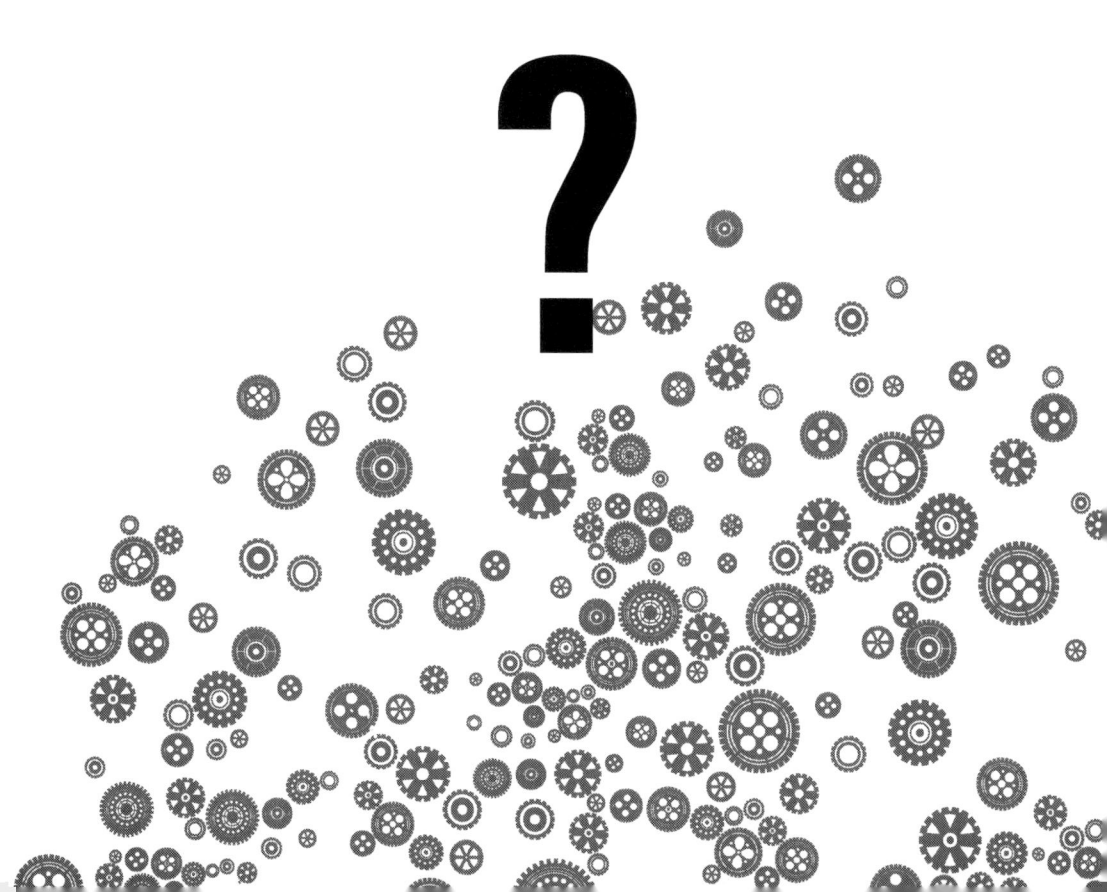

If you said 'Why …?' or 'How …?' you would be like the many school staff I have asked this same question to over recent years. And, like them, you would be wrong.

The one question that is always active in our children's subconscious minds is:

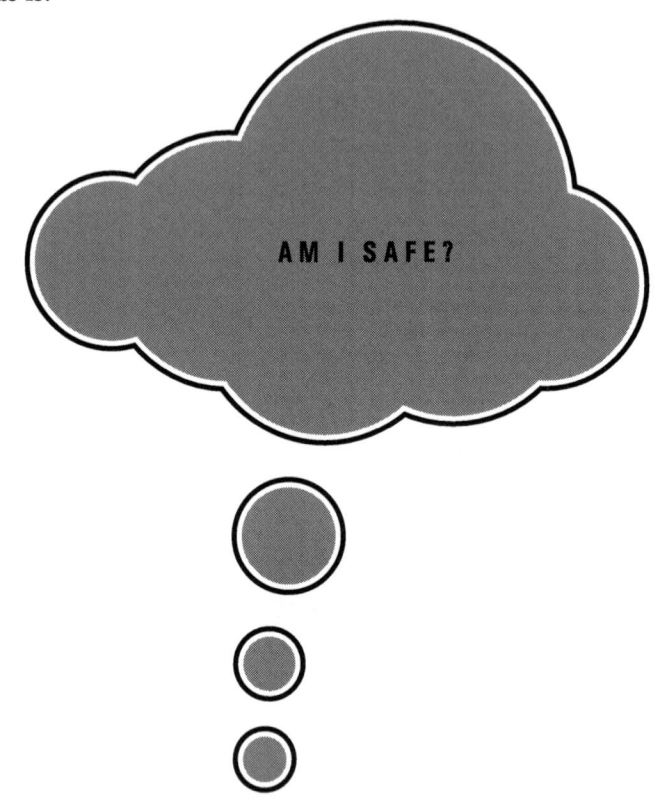

AM I SAFE?

Depending on where a child is, what is happening around them, and who they are with, the answer can change in a heartbeat. Because it is a question held in the subconscious, it is unlikely that a child would ever give you that answer out loud if you were to ask them. And yet, sure enough, should anything happen to make them feel *un*safe, their nervous system will respond instantly.

Dr Porges explains that children are constantly taking in information to answer this million-dollar question. He calls it the process of 'neuroception', and he defines it like this:

> Neuroception, distinct from perception ... is detection without awareness. It is the subconscious process whereby the nervous system, through processing sensory information, then works out via neural circuits if a person or experience is safe/dangerous/life-threatening.
> *Dr Stephen Porges*

So, what does this all mean for understanding children and bringing the best out of them? How does this help the teacher in a classroom trying to get a new learning point across? How is it relevant for a parent trying to deal with an upset child (maybe because they didn't understand the new learning point at school, and 'forgot' to bring home their homework on it)?

To answer these questions, there is something important we need to understand about children and how they decide whether they can come to us when they are struggling or need to stay away, to find their own solutions (which may include denial or avoidance) and 'tough it out' on their own.

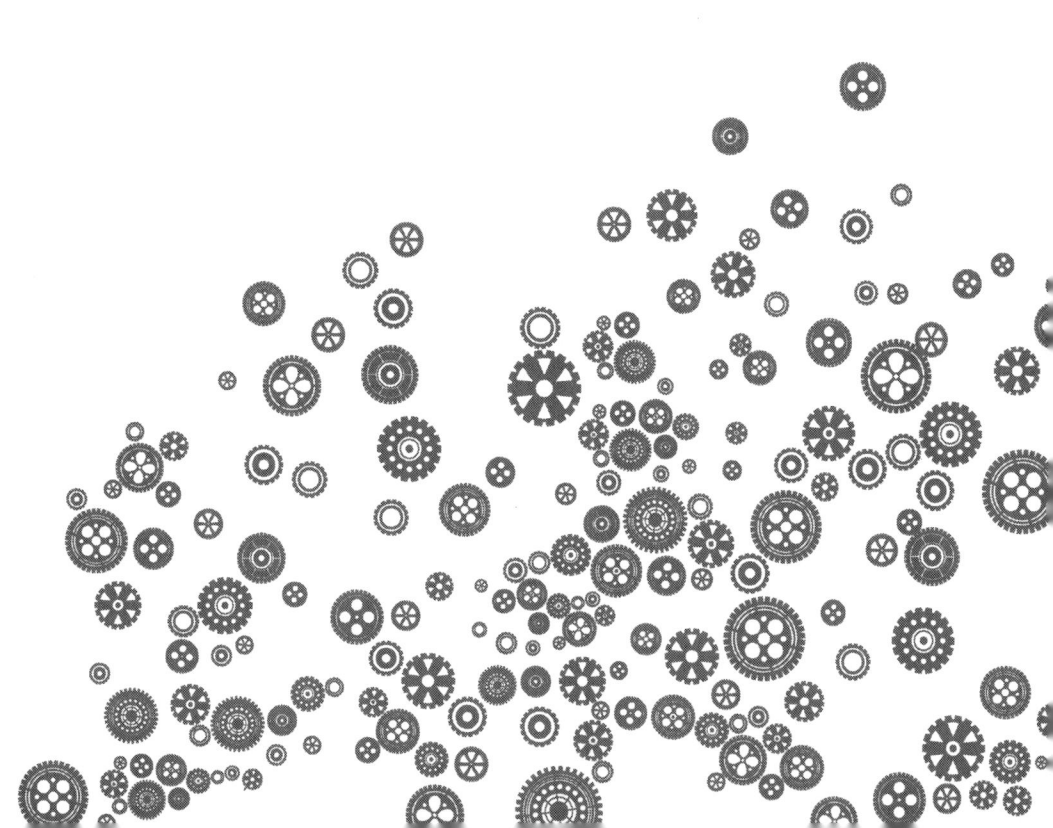

5

Learning From The Animals

From the moment they are born, children need adults. We are their source of *life*. We are the providers of food, warmth, cleaning, connection and protection. They know instinctively that their key adult is there to take care of them and keep them safe. In this way they are like so many other little ones in the animal kingdom.

If mummy bear is happily playing with her cubs one minute, and the next she gets a scent of wolf on the breeze, she will stop playing. She will look about, maybe getting up on her haunches, using her ears and nose as well as her eyes, to try and locate the danger. The cubs may not know exactly what she is doing, but her change in attention, behaviour, breathing and muscle tightness lets them know she is doing something important; this is serious. They will stick close by her until she relaxes again once the threat has gone, or she moves them to their den for protection. When they are with her, the little cubs take their cue of how safe they are from mummy bear. Children do the same.

My dog on the drive

It was the first Monday of the new school year – a day that most children across the country were truly thankful for, because they got one more day to stay at home, while knowing all their teachers were already back at school!

I was booked to deliver training to the entire staff team at a large primary school for their INSET teacher training day. My dog was booked into his favourite dog-sitter and his bed and dinner were in the car, ready to go. I popped his lead on and we walked outside. He came with me happily out of the front door, and only as I opened the back of the car did he stop moving. I encouraged him to get in. Nothing. I showed him the treats he would get, and his favourite squeaky toys. Nothing. He turned his handsome but wilful head and looked away from the car. I became more emphatic in my encouragement. Nothing. This was not like him. He usually got into the car in no time – and if this went on much longer, I would be late dropping him off at his dog-sitter.

OK, I decided, I would nip this in the bud and change tack to the 'no messing, I mean it' approach. Firmer tone, the one-finger point, "get in". Still nothing.

I noticed I was getting annoyed with him now. He needed to get in, and now! I had to get him dropped off, come back home, grab a shower, load the car with my training resources and then go and deliver my training. He didn't seem to care.

I know he is a sensitive boy, and my getting louder and shouting at him would not have got us anywhere. So I changed tack again. I took a deep breath and just thought to myself, 'OK, buddy boy, I will wait. You take your time. You know what you need to do; we both know you can do it. I'll just wait.'

My dog, the mind-reader, instantly responded by sitting his golden furry bottom down on the drive and looking up at me with his deep-brown, sensitive, loyal eyes! If he could have spoken, it would have been: "Yes, I hear you, you are waiting, and I'm gonna wait with you".

I made one trip back inside the house to find his best chew toy and smother it in a teaspoon of peanut butter before bringing him and it back outside, and this was the in-the-moment distraction he needed to know that something good was happening. He jumped into the car, got stuck in to his treat, and we were off.

To an observer, that wasn't his finest hour. He didn't do well. He didn't behave the way he should have, the way he could, or the way I asked and then told him to.

It would be really easy to put all the focus on him, and chastise him for his behaviour, his disobedience.

But that wouldn't be fair.

The truth was, I was the bigger part of what was happening on my drive. I was busy telling myself I was fine – it was just another piece of training, like I had done so many times before. He, however, could tell I was nervous. He would have been able to smell my stress. My body was tight, I was rushing, I probably sounded different, and the tension in my facial muscles wouldn't have been lost on him.

He didn't know the 'change' in me was only about going to deliver some new training to a large staff team. He didn't know that I knew I would be OK, and he was actually going to have a great day himself. No. He could just sense my nervousness – my fear. When animals sense fear in those closest to them, they often stay close. The survival instinct (in this type of moment for dogs, bear cubs and some children) says we stand a better chance if we are together. He was not going to leave me – his nervous, focused, tense, I've-got-a-big-day-ahead 'parent' – to go through it alone.

As I reflected on what had happened on the drive, it only made sense as I became honest about *my* emotional and physical state and admitted my nervousness. When I acknowledged that I was, in fact, *really* nervous about delivering this new training for the first time, I could understand his dog's subconscious process: 'my human is not OK; that means things are not OK, which means danger, which means I'm not OK ... which means I need to stay safe and stick close by her – and doing that is more important than doing what I'm told!'

And this is the thing. As adults we cannot write ourselves out of the stories of the children around us. Children can detect when the adult they are with is not 'OK', and it affects them. This is the neuroception that Dr Porges speaks about. Sometimes they respond by trying to stay close. At other times, like Lisa's daughters, they try to stay away. Children do not exist in isolation, whatever the state of the 'relationship' we *feel* we have – they do relate to us. Day by day, in both the significant and the unassuming moments, we are part of their story. If the children around us are behaving in ways that are not their best selves when we are with them, then to begin really understanding what is going on with them we can start by looking at ourselves and seeing what part we might have played in that.

6

Getting Perspective

Before we go any further, we need to clarify something. You may well be thinking: 'Wait a minute! Is that really true? Is how safe a child feels *all* dependent on the adult they are with? Is it true that how a child is behaving is *all* because of me?' If that resonates with your thoughts, then this section is especially for you.

In short, the quick answer is no. There are four main areas that we need to consider if we want to really understand what factors may be affecting a child and their level of emotional and physical safety in any particular, present moment: what's going on in the vicinity around them; the way they are communicated with; their own internal environment; and the 'state' of the person they are with.

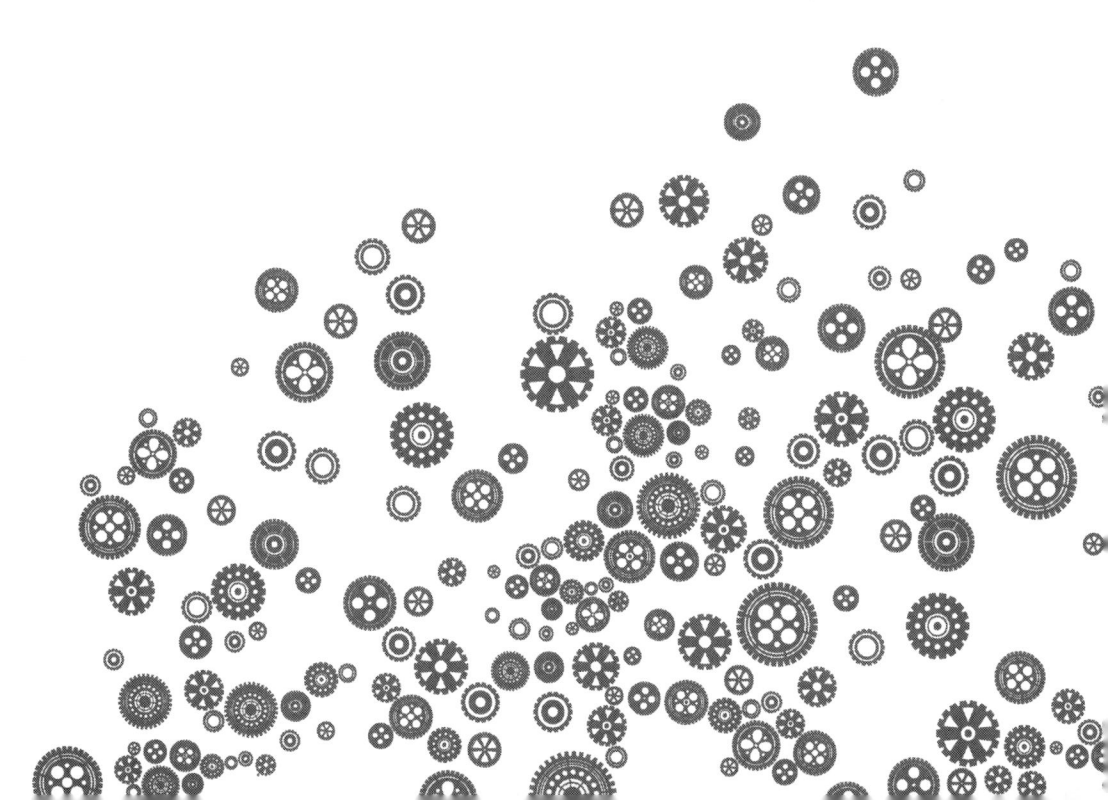

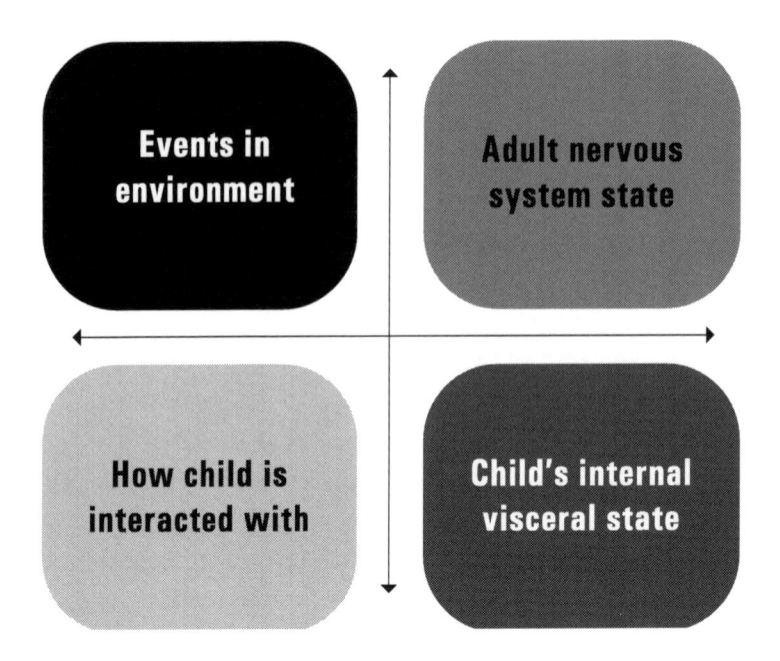

Events in environment	**Adult nervous system state**
How child is interacted with	**Child's internal visceral state**

Four areas for assessing safety

1. The environment

A peaceful beach where a child is happily playing in the sand; piling onto one bed or sofa for snuggles with their special people; playing and making a mighty mess; and 'creating' when they are surrounded by people who are happy with what's going on, and they know it is OK to express themselves freely. These are all examples of environments that are more likely to feel safe to a child.

A busy park where a big, barking dog is bounding towards them; sitting a test at school; and being anywhere where adults are shouting, whether they are drunk, celebrating a sports win or just arguing, are all likely to result in a child feeling less safe, and aware of the potential danger they are in.

As adults, while we may have a good idea, we cannot assume that we can predict the type of environment that will have one child feeling safe and another under threat. Fireworks would be one example; art lessons, particular sounds, PE, music, smells, playtime, dinner-time and home time are others. Some children feel their safest environment is home;

others relax when they get to the predictability and routine of school on a Monday morning. Some children *love* their bedrooms, while for others it is not a safe environment to be in.

> I will never forget one lad telling me his favourite time at school – the time he felt safest was during lockdown. For this English school, lockdown meant one of the students in the school was really struggling, probably no longer contained within their classroom, and probably embarking on an angry rampage around the school. In this particular school, it was not an unusual occurrence. This was a time when the teaching staff were aware of the enormity of the situation, and the potential risk of harm to this student, to others and/or to property.
>
> With many adults feeling less safe, how was it that this boy said 'lockdown' was the best time? His reasons were simple. The classroom door was locked – the child in the corridors couldn't get in. The lights (which gave him a headache) were turned off. Everyone had to be silent (it was the *only* time his 'ears got a break all day'). However, the biggest bonus was that no one was allowed to move out of their seats. During normal class activities, there were children who would be up and out of their seats and often over to hassle him at his desk. When moving around wasn't allowed, he was safe.

Lighting, sounds, movement and interior design are often forgotten in terms of their impact on many children. There is a fine line between stimulation and overstimulation; between awareness and overwhelm. Fire alarms, pneumatic drills, smoke alarms and emergency services sirens are all designed to catch our attention and make us aware of them – to put us on alert. Watch how your adult heart rate goes up when you next hear that screeching coming up behind you and catch the first glimpse of those blue lights flashing in your rear-view mirror. The alert physiology is the same – if not more so – for children.

2. The way the child is communicated with
No one likes being shouted at or snapped at. No one really enjoys being told what to do. No one enjoys feeling intimidated. No one brings out

their best when they are feeling forced, manipulated or exploited.

The *way* we communicate with children can have an incredible impact – for good or ill. It is very common that the voices children hear in their heads when they are older – the voices that are referred to as 'self-talk' – speak words the child first heard when they were little. For many adults, how to be with and speak to a child to really bring out their best does not come naturally. Many adults didn't get the benefit of being spoken to in ways that honoured them when *they* were children. However, the good news is that these skills are easy to learn and practise. One of my favourite ways to improve the bond between a child and an adult – when supporting a parent, carer or someone at school – is by helping the grown-up grow new skills. However much we can already do, there is always something more to learn! An experienced senior primary school teacher sent the following email the day after going on some communication skills training:

> In terms of the session last night, it made me reflect on things that I do/say and my practice in general. I had already started trying different techniques you've suggested in the past, but even last night I realised that things still needed changing more. This afternoon in my class was classic. ... A child was constantly trying to share his ideas during a P4C discussion and dominate the class. Previously I may have reminded him of the 'shouting out' rules (and a few minutes later he would have done it again) but today I did the 'your opinion is really valuable to us and we all want to hear what you have to say so could you wait until it's your turn so we can all listen to just you?' He did, and we had a really successful afternoon. At about 1.30 pm today he had said he wanted to go home, at 3.20 pm he was saying 'do I have to go home?'.

When a child feels respected and safe with the interaction they are having with you, they will share more of their thoughts and feelings with you, and to a greater level of honesty. However, if they don't feel totally comfortable (with you or the environment), then the superficial or monosyllabic responses are more likely. The way an adult chooses to communicate with a child can change the entire relationship. It is one of the quickest and simplest ways to change the atmosphere in a home or classroom.

3. The child's internal environment

Something that is little appreciated when we are considering children's behaviour is the incredible connection between our brain and our body. Stephen Porges explains that, during the process of neuroception, as well as taking in external information from our senses, our brain also receives information from *within the body* about what's going on and what that means for our safety.

The internal 'scan' is significant. Very simply put, if the brain receives information that, for example, muscles are tight, then the message the brain gets is 'muscles are tight'. The brain knows that tight muscles are one of the indicators of not being safe – it's what happens when danger is near. Increased heart rate and quicker breathing are just two more of the many signals that something is not OK. Fever, pain or other physical illness are also indicators that all is not well, or safe, internally and can activate the same neurophysiological changes.

Stress prevents feeling safe

We will look at other physiological responses to not being safe in a later chapter. For now, let's just appreciate that any children who are continually experiencing tight muscles, increased heart rate and more shallow breathing will struggle to feel safe because their body is sending to their subconscious brain messages to the contrary. Learning to release tension, be able to relax muscles and slow down breathing and heart rate is important for children and adults alike. My experience, from having worked in this area for over 15 years, is that for some people it is easier said than done. If it does not come naturally, then it can really help to work with a qualified body-aware provider and go at a pace that feels OK to you/your child (some suggested links are provided at the end of the book). For anyone, adult or child, who has experienced trauma or prolonged periods of high stress, tension or anxiety in the past, this can be a bigger challenge – but still one that it is absolutely possible to overcome given the right tools, techniques, support and timing.

There are many ways to help the body temporarily relax a bit more. There are also some incredible ways to help release long-held patterns of deep tension, which make 'relaxed' more of an everyday experience rather than a place to visit or go to on vacation now and again. Maybe you can imagine the increased sense of being 'safe in my body' when long-held tension has gone from muscles, breathing is organically slower and deeper, and a smile is more frequently found loitering in the mouth and eyes?

Essential elements
Ensuring that a child is drinking enough water can be crucially important in helping their body function at its best.

Our bodies were designed to function on a wide range of essential elements. Water is one; a wide spectrum of micronutrients is another. Sadly, a complete balance of antioxidants, vitamins and minerals is missing from the diets of the vast majority of adults and children across the world. Without optimum levels of these micronutrients resourcing cells to do their various jobs, our cells – and therefore our muscles and bodies – struggle to function in an optimal state.

A top-quality magnesium nutritional supplement can help tight muscles to relax, and including it with a balance of other essential micronutrients can be one way to help change the 'tight-unsafe' story from the inside out.

> Max was a four-year-old who had already been diagnosed with non-verbal autism. He seemed happy at home with his core family but found trips out in his pushchair too much. As is so common for autistic children, his body was tight and tense, and he never made eye contact. His mum was desperate.
>
> She was an astute woman and knew that his diet of ham, crisps, crackers and the occasional yogurt was not going to help his body or brain to thrive. Getting a complete balance of micronutrients into Max daily was an attempt to do something to change this picture, which felt – like his taste-buds – set in stone. She was careful to use high-quality products that were independently verified to actually deliver to the body

what they said on the label. Max's mum knew enough to know that supplements were not all created equal, and she couldn't risk giving Max anything that wasn't of the highest quality.

It was complete joy, relief and gratitude that came through her tears down the telephone a few weeks later. She admitted to having been sceptical, and this was certainly not a done deal, but crushing the micronutrients into his yogurt had worked to get them inside him happily and she couldn't believe how her boy was changing. The phrase that stuck with me from our long conversation was "he seems more peaceful. He seems happier in himself. He even seems more relaxed." She, too, felt able to relax more now, knowing that, for now at least, his body was getting a broad spectrum of the essential micronutrients it needed to function, and to deal with the day-by-day impact of stress that 'life' was for him. From this point, they were able to move forward into other ways of helping him thrive.

Everybody knows that omega oils are critical for brain function. So for a child who is having trouble concentrating, there is a chance that – as well as cleaning up the food that is going into their mouths on a daily basis and reducing their intake of chemicals and sugars etc. – adding a simple daily intake of quality omega oils can help to give their brain the resources it was designed to function with. I have seen the benefits of this for so many children. The official research is proving this, over and over again.

4. The person they are with

As you can see, there are many indicators that keep a child's subconscious brain busy answering the question "am I safe right now?".

The final factor is the relational one – person-to-person. If a child doesn't feel safe around an adult, they very rarely have the words or cognitive function – let alone the confidence or courage – to be able to say to the grown-up, "I don't feel safe because I don't feel *you* are safe". Instead, their body just responds, and their behaviour reacts: fighting, crying, shouting, arguing, hitting, running or going into a state of silent shut-down. What happens to children when they exhibit this behaviour? Often they get disciplined. Whether this means a timeout, a naughty step, a loss of toys, treats or favourite activities, moving down the traffic lights, a red card, a previously earned token taken out of the jar, or other warning … they are made to pay for the way their body just responded to an ungrounded, and therefore unsafe, adult body.

Even if we are not the trigger for a child not feeling safe, the level of 'safety' and grounded-ness we are in will affect how much we are able to support them. Our own level of stress will determine how effective we can be (or not) in helping the child to calm and find safety again. I have lost count of the situations in which this has played out in schools and homes. Imagine a child is struggling with a piece of (home)work, maybe also because they have a fear of failure or they fear the consequences that will come if they get it wrong. They do not feel safe enough with the adult in the room (who happens to have their own significant stress story going on) to use them as a resource. They do not ask for help. Instead they feel alone with their struggle and will 'behave' their way to safety – through creating a battle, getting away or shutting down. I have had the privilege of helping many parents discover their own story as a major piece in the puzzle of their child's behaviour. We can busy ourselves with all the 'just-focus-on-the-now' energy we can muster to hold in, deny or suppress how we still feel about the things that happened to us in the past. But it is when we realise that the tension in us is not hidden from the kids around us that we can start to ask ourselves if their behaviour is almost like a barometer for our own stress levels, our internal, unexpressed fear or held-in anger.

Happy mummy, happy babies …

Tracey was a mum of three little ones. She had gone through a really demanding divorce and was left picking up the pieces of her life, with her young children at the centre. Today had been hard. She'd had a phone call from a lawyer and it hadn't gone well. She was spoken to abruptly, and hearing 'that tone' again had triggered her. She felt angry and she felt vulnerable. Her body got tight, she struggled to keep breathing and she feared the man on the other end would be able to hear her heart beating, it was suddenly so loud. She started shaking, with the phone still held to her head. Somehow she held it together long enough to end the conversation and get off the phone. She reversed the two steps into the chair in the corner of her kitchen, sat down and cried. With one child upstairs creating new worlds with his Lego and the other two playing in the lounge, she stifled the noises she really wanted to release. She couldn't go there. She didn't want to upset her kids, and it was nearly their bedtime. She just needed to make it through …

As best she could, she pulled the emotions back inside and blew her nose. She didn't even notice the rest of her body. She just needed her face to look 'normal'. The two in the lounge started crying. More emotion. Her girls had seen something on TV that scared them and now, unusually, they wouldn't let her comfort them. She made tea, hoping it would be a good distraction, and then immediately started on the bath/bed routine. Things went from bad to worse. She normally enjoyed this time of day with her tribe. Tonight she just had to get through and was counting the minutes. They wouldn't calm, and they wouldn't settle. They knew something was up. They couldn't know what or why, they just knew. Their tears were their only way to communicate their knowing that things were different, that their 'mummy bear' was different – and that made *them* feel … different. It made them feel confused andscared.

The role an adult's stress level plays – or, more precisely, *the impact on a child of the amount of activation in the adult's nervous system* – is very rarely understood or appreciated. If we want to really understand children, unravel the mystery of their behaviour, support them and bring out the best in them, then we need to see ourselves as a crucial part of the picture. Rather than disabling us by piling on guilt or shame, if we understand this and see it play out in our own stories, it brings us power. There is something we have clarity on and we can make a change. That we are always part of our children's behaviour puzzle is, in fact, a concept so crucial that it needed to be the main theme of this whole book!

7

Neuroception In The Movies

To use our nervous system, our body, to help calm down a child when they are upset, is called *co-regulation*. This cannot and will not happen if the child doesn't feel safe with us at that time. Neither can it happen if our nervous system is more activated/stressed than theirs. We cannot kid ourselves – a child's neuroception is a powerful, functioning, living resource. They want to be *safe* and, no matter what we may tell them with our words, they have their own life-sustaining instinct telling them whether we, in our body, right at that moment, can help them get there or not.

It is important that we understand that we are not talking about a simple Yes/No answer to the question of a child's personal sense of safety:

Am I safe? Yes – then everything is fine.

Am I safe? No – then I do X, Y or Z.

It is, not surprisingly, a 'bit' more complex than that!

Remember that the definition of neuroception (see page 19) talks about children working out if they are:

1) safe
2) in danger, or
3) their life is threatened.

There are three possible options, and the behaviours that come with each are significantly different. Each phase is actually driven by a different neurophysiological 'system' or 'set-up' in the brain and body. We will break these down, so we can understand the differences of each in a further section. For now, here it is in a diagram.

Neuroception In The Movies | 33

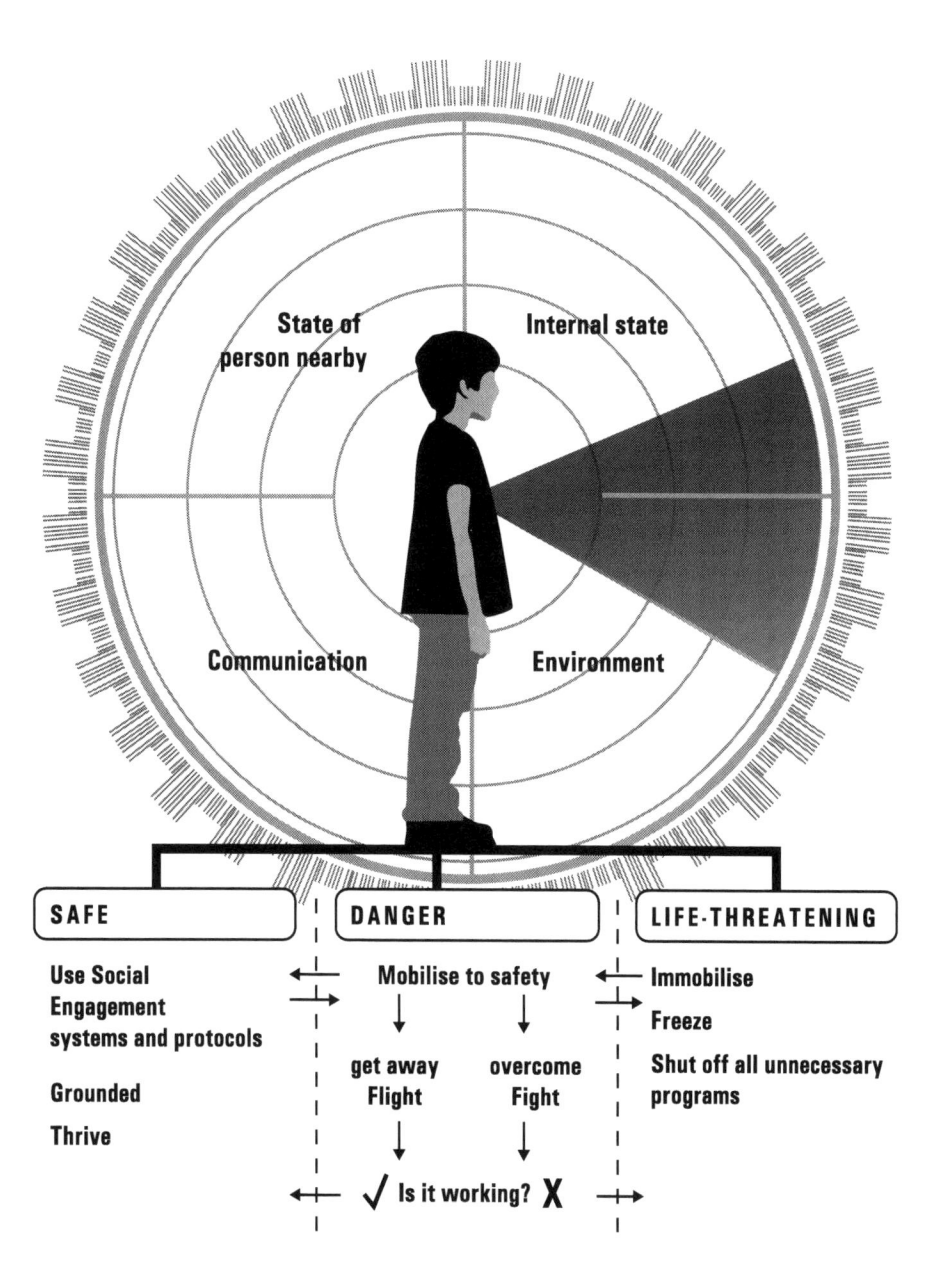

Radar diagram quadrants: State of person nearby | Internal state | Communication | Environment

SAFE	DANGER	LIFE-THREATENING
Use Social Engagement systems and protocols	← Mobilise to safety ←	← Immobilise
	↓ ↓	Freeze
Grounded	get away / overcome	Shut off all unnecessary programs
Thrive	Flight / Fight	
	↓ ↓	
	✓ Is it working? ✗ →	

Neuroception and the stages of survival

Obviously, real life never feels like it fits into neat diagrams; however, it is amazing how accurately this one describes the process that children go through every day. If we dig a bit deeper into the neuroscience and neurophysiology, we can understand this more, and we can do it in a way that is easy to relate to! Let's go to the movies.

Captain Phillips

Neuroception and the process, behaviours and stages of survival were powerfully represented in a film I saw recently. The 2013 film *Captain Phillips*, starring Tom Hanks, is a dramatic retelling of a true story. In 2009 an American container ship, MV *Maersk Alabama*, was passing the coast of Somalia when it was attacked by Somali pirates. I am aware that there is some controversy over the film's portrayal of Captain Phillips as a hero (the real crew said he was far from it, and actually was the one who put the ship in danger in the first place). I don't know all the details, and only have the film to go on. Well, the first half, actually, as I didn't make it through to the end – it created too much sustained tension for me (or my body) to 'enjoy' for two and a quarter hours straight! However, the bit I saw is relevant for us now.

For the *Maersk Alabama*, it was business as usual. Although everyone knew the waters off the coast of Somalia were a risky place to be, the weather was good, the crew were working, taking breaks, eating, drinking and sleeping, and the atmosphere was relaxed. The ship's internal systems – engine pressure, temperature etc. – were being monitored (*N:* checking for safety from internal body sources like heart rate, breathing rate, muscle tension etc.) and everything was ticking over nicely. The radar was checked regularly, and officers frequently used binoculars to scan the surrounding area from the bridge and stern (*N:* using senses in checking for safety from 'environment'). The horizon was clear, with no visible threat anywhere.

Two little spots appearing on the radar caught the attention of the captain. They were quickly identified as two small boats loaded with Somali pirates. They had guns and, even though the ship dwarfed them, it appeared that they were headed straight for the **Maersk Alabama**.

The captain ordered the crew to assume their positions in the muster stations – this was not a drill; there was now imminent danger (*N:* moving from social engagement 'safe' to threatened 'danger' state).

He ordered a slight change of course (*N:* first attempt to mobilise and move away from the threat (flight)). Just five degrees to port would be enough to see if the spots on the radar were going to follow. The spots tracked the ship exactly. It was being chased, and the enemy, albeit in tiny high-speed fishing boats, were gaining on it.

Captain Phillips ordered the engines to push harder and harder (*N:* second attempt to mobilise and move away from the threat). The spots on the radar moved faster, getting closer, and could be clearly seen through his binoculars. It was only a matter of minutes before they would be visible to the naked eye.

Moving away (flight) didn't work. The threat was still there – the danger still imminent. It was time for different tactics. The captain ordered another slight change of direction, combined with a further increase in speed, with the aim of creating a much bigger wake behind his vessel (*N:* changing survival approach from flight to fight tactic no. 1). In the way a dog growls, snarls and bares his teeth before his attack, surely the increased waves behind the *Maersk Alabama* would show the ship's power to the small, battered, speeding boats? It worked – for one boat, whose crew took the warning and decided these waves were too much for them. If they continued pushing on through, it was likely they'd be capsized very soon. They pulled back and headed back to shore. There was now just one relentless dot getting closer and closer to the centre of the radar screen … until it suddenly stopped moving. The crew of the *Maersk Alabama* didn't know that the pirates' engine had cut out, leaving them stranded. The gap between the vessels gradually increased again, but the *Maersk Alabama* crew stayed vigilant. They were not able to return to a relaxed state of safety yet; they knew pirates, and they were a determined, resilient foe. While they stayed in these waters, threat remained.

Maintaining a state of high alert on the ship proved to be wise, as the next morning the larger pirate boat was back and gaining on them again. The *Maersk Alabama* was a container ship, not a vessel of war. It was not fitted with guns or cannon. The major 'weapon' on board with which to 'fight' was the system of firefighting water jets located all around the perimeter of the ship. On the captain's command, water began gushing out of each jet (*N:* fight tactic no. 2). Would this serve to deter or even capsize the resolute pirates? No. They found a gap large enough to sneak their boat through and, once behind the pounding jets, they continued the short distance to the ship's hull, unhindered.

The last resource in the ship's 'arsenal' (N: fight tactic no. 3) was a desperate, creative (mis)use of flares. One by one, the flares that were designed to burn brightly and draw attention to a vessel in distress were activated and, once flaming intensely, were launched like miniature scud missiles at the pirates' boat, each one missing by a fraction.

The pirates, set on their mission to use this huge American ship to extort the money they wanted, were not giving up. They spotted a place to connect their ladder to the hull and, one by one, with military-issue guns strapped to their backs, began climbing up and boarding the ship.

The captain, realising that the threat level had just increased significantly, had a few moments before the pirates were smashing their way to where he was located, on the bridge – the control hub of the ship. He changed tactics again (N: moving into the state of overwhelm and 'life-threatening'), ordering the crew to hiding places in the engine room in the bowels of the ship. Doors were locked. He ordered the engines be shut off, together with all the electricity, and other power sources. To all intents and purposes, the ship would now appear 'dead in the water' (N: total immobilisation (freeze)).

Mission: Staying alive

Whatever our age, whatever we might think, our biggest goal is to stay alive. From the day we arrive on this earth until the day we leave it, we go through this same process over and over again, every day. Every time our subconscious process picks up a hint of danger, our nervous system reacts, and our body and behaviour respond. We either move away from the threat or towards it to deal with it, or – just like the *Maersk Alabama* – if these approaches haven't helped us, we shut down.

However, it is not all one-way. If, like a fugitive on the run, we determine we have used our flight system enough, and that we are far enough away from the threat, we can reassess the danger level and, if it has gone down, our nervous system will recalibrate. If we feel completely free from threat, our state of safety can resume once again and will set in operation our brain-body system, which Stephen Porges calls our Social Engagement System.

What do you notice?

It is great to be learning about survival patterns with movies involving boats and pirates, but what is really going to help you is to consider when you see this playing out with your children. Here are a few questions for you to ask yourself – and jot down your thoughts if it helps give you clarity.

- When the children you care about feel safe, who are they? What words would you use to describe them? What can they do that is different to when they don't feel safe?
- Does this child have a greater tendency towards 'fight' or to 'flight'?
- What kind of thing do you notice this child does when they are going into 'fight' or 'flight'? Sometimes it is not as obvious as kicking or hitting, or running away.
- Does this child seem like they are shutting down? What do you notice and what are the things that seem to trigger them into this state?

NB If you find it hard to know who this child is when they are completely safe, it may be because you haven't seen this yet. It is worth considering the possibility that you have never seen a particular child feel completely safe. It may be more as if they are stuck in a loop between danger and life-threatening states. If this is the case, don't worry – stay with me and we will talk more about this later.

8

It's Not Just The Children

It was about 30 minutes into my second meeting with this mum. We had covered a lot of ground together the previous time, and to her credit she had tried out many of the suggestions I had given her and her partner. They had been desperate to understand their daughter better, and the realisations of what they were doing that were making life even harder for her had come thick and fast when we last met. They were committed, though. They had spent the last two weeks trying out different approaches and meeting their daughter with appropriate understanding instead of frustration. So this, our second meeting, was largely a celebration. It was wonderful to hear how things were changing at home, to honour the effort they were putting in and to celebrate the positive impact they were already having. I was so proud of this lady and the effort she was putting in to becoming even more the mum her daughter needed.

The atmosphere was light; we were both relaxed. There had been many smiles, laughter, and 'hoorays' celebrating their progress. We shared lots of great eye contact and both of us were feeling comfortable in the other's presence.

Then she mentioned how mealtimes were still sometimes tricky. I asked her what she would say when her daughter was struggling at the table. And she told me. She told me like it was tea-time and I was across the table from her.

Instantly my body became tight. I felt sick, and moved backwards in my chair. My heart beat fast and loud. I felt small, my face flushed, and I wanted to get out.

Why?

Here we were, two grown adults having a conversation about a little girl and what happened at mealtimes. We were on the same side, but suddenly in these moments, as this mum re-enacted what she said to her daughter at the table, and how she said it, I felt threatened.

The actual words she used are not important. What was significant was how, in an instant, I had gone from feeling very comfortable with her, operating in my 'social engagement system', to not feeling at all safe and wanting to get out (flight). Her energy had suddenly changed and, although she hadn't touched me, I experienced her frustration with full force from her body. She had spoken loudly and fast. She had moved up and forwards in her chair and gestured emphatically with her hand. Her words were clipped and suddenly it felt like I was across the table from a tyrant. My 'head' knew I was still physically safe. My nervous system, however, had picked up on the messages from her verbal and non-verbal communication and perceived that I was in danger and needed to get away. My body was where our breakthrough lesson was.

It is not just children who live by the process of neuroception.

I was able to notice what had happened in me, inside my body, inside my nervous system, and we talked about it. We were able to use my experience to help her. I shared with this mum that, even though I knew she wasn't talking to me, her tone, the speed of her words and the aggressive energy behind what she said had made me, a grown-up, feel overwhelmed. If I had been a little girl on the receiving end of that energy from my mum, I know my nervous system would respond just the same and I would be very scared.

This honourable mum was humble, open and able to receive what I shared with her. She had felt a change inside her system, too (going from calm into an angry 'fight' energy). She said that she had moments like this with her partner, too, and at work. To her complete credit, she took this moment of self-realisation and honesty, and chose to grow. This mum chose to become aware of herself. She realised that, in order to fulfil her desire to keep helping her daughter, she now actually needed to focus on helping herself.

SECTION 2

UNDERSTANDING SURVIVAL

The rules of survival never change, whether you're in a
desert or in an arena.

Bear Grylls

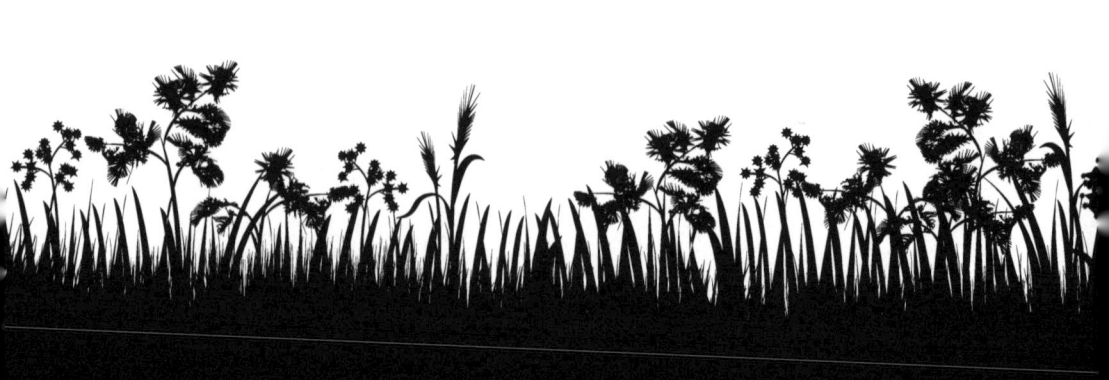

9

F's For Survival

Most people have heard of the three common survival states. If we feel that something is threatening to us, most people know their 'F' words! More precisely, they have heard of the three F's: Fight, Flight and Freeze.

It can really help us to understand more about these states. When we can get our heads around thriving versus surviving, we will better understand our children and ourselves and how to navigate the relationships between us.

Let us invest some time together in really understanding the differences that occur in our brains and bodies, what we can and can't do, what we will and won't do, how we behave, and how we see ourselves and the world around us when we are in these different states.

Unlike the common view that these three states are all equal options we are faced with, we will understand that Fight and Flight are both rooted in trying to mobilise or move ourselves towards or away from the danger. Freeze is something we only go to if neither of the others has worked, and is our last-ditch attempt at surviving. It shows us that things have got really serious.

Our mobilising (movement) behaviours and our shut-down, immobilising state are made clearer to us when we see how different they are to our social engagement – the 'I *am* safe' state. So, let's start there. Let's start by really understanding what it means to be safe. What it means to thrive.

10

Social Engagement System

General state: 'I am safe'

Nothing bad is happening

Nothing bad is going to happen

I can thrive

Nervous system: My parasympathetic nervous system is dominant
My ventral vagus nerve/myelinated vagus nerve is in charge and happily sending information from my brain to my gut and from my gut and muscles back to my brain. It also keeps the flow of energy moving from my brainstem through one of its branches into my heart, and through another into the nerves in my eyes, facial muscles and middle ear

Eyes
My eyes work (as well as they are able)

I can make eye contact

I can read other people well – I can pick up small nuances in their tone of voice and muscle tension, and understand what they are really thinking

My face moves with different emotions as I feel them

I can smile with my eyes

Hearing

My ears work well and can hear a wide range of sound frequencies

I can filter out background noises

I can focus in on noises I want to pay attention to (a friend speaking in a noisy place like a café, dinner hall or playground; a teacher or boss speaking in a noisy room)

I hear what people are saying to me

I can listen and process what is being said

I can follow instructions

Body

My heart rate is steady

My breathing is regular, and I can breathe deeply from my abdomen

My appetite is working well – I know when I am hungry and respond to it

My digestive system is functioning well

I can go to the toilet easily and regularly, and notice when I need to

I sleep well

My immune system works well

I can notice my body on the inside. I can feel when my muscles are tight, and relax them

neocortex

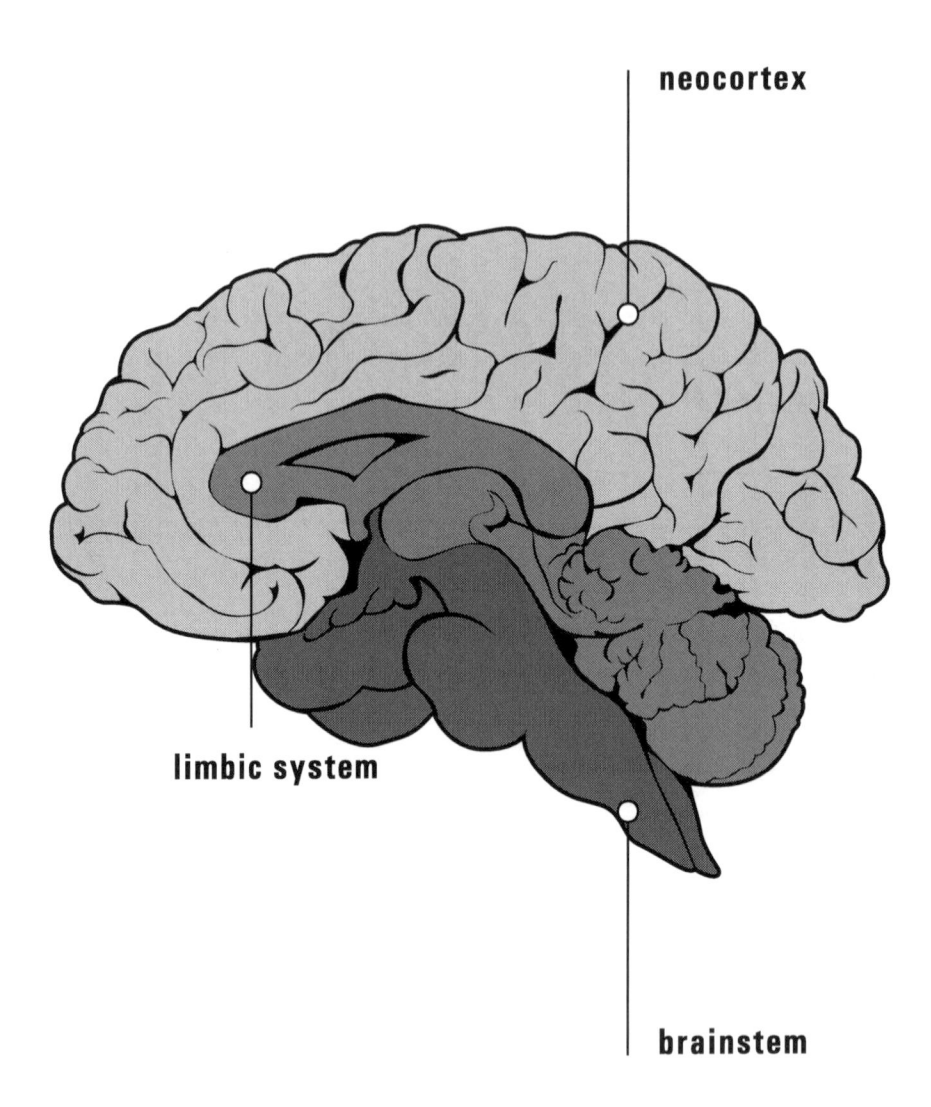

limbic system

brainstem

All working well

Brain

My neocortex is working well. This is the part of my brain that helps me do all the things humans can – plan, organise, solve tricky problems and even speak!

I can think, make ('good') choices and reason (at the level for my emotional age)

Interactions

I am happy to connect with others – it feels safe to do so

I pick up on jokes and humour

I can tell easily if people are lying

I read a blank face as a blank face – it is neutral to me, and I can try to engage with the person and see if they will connect with me

I can stick around when others are upset, angry or anxious. I can consider options about whether they are upset because of me or something else

I can access and develop empathy

Life view

I see the world as a (generally) good place to be

I have an open posture and attitude to life

I can explore, expand and increase the 'size' of my life by going to new places and learning and doing new things

I can take risks

I can be creative

I can feel my own body sensations

I can feel the parts of me that are connecting to something else

I am aware of and can connect with my feelings, my body, my surroundings and others

I am open to building a bond with others

I am prepared to gradually share more information about me, as I feel I want to

I am 'grounded'

I can thrive!

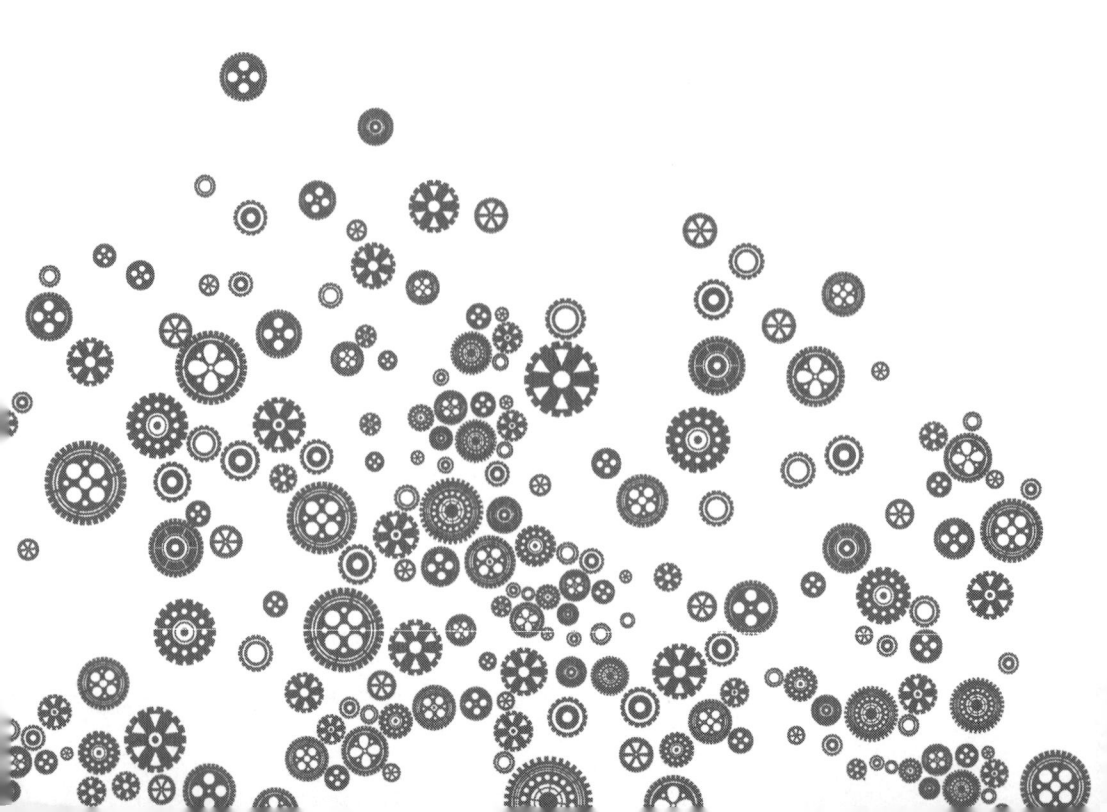

11

Mobilisation/Defence

General state: 'I'm not safe'

    It is dangerous

    Something bad might happen

Nervous system: My sympathetic nervous system is dominant

My myelinated vagus nerve has shut off and taken with it all the functions it carries out – these are not needed when I need to prioritise surviving

Eyes
My eyes narrow

I look around – I keep alert to locating danger

My eyebrows change position

My pupils dilate to let in more light and help improve my sight to keep my optical information coming in well

My eyesight changes

My field of vision gets narrower (tunnel vision)

Hearing

My hearing changes – I can no longer hear all frequencies

I can hear predominantly low frequencies as my middle ear has changed and I am focused on listening out for threats in the low frequencies

I cannot hear everything you are saying

I cannot understand what you are saying at my normal processing speed, if at all

I cannot sift out background noise in a classroom, playground, restaurant, shopping centre or anywhere busy

I feel like my hearing has become more sensitive and everything seems louder now

Body

The change in the part of my nervous system operating me has triggered my adrenal glands to go to work and release the hormones I need to survive

My body is pumping with adrenaline – and noradrenaline and cortisol too, if I stay like this a long time

My heart rate is fast

Blood gets diverted to my major muscle groups

My breathing is faster and shallow – just in the top of my lungs

I am ready to move – I need to defend myself

I engage my 'fight' or 'flight' mode

Fight: I become argumentative

> I am aggressive
>
> I speak loudly
>
> I shout more readily
>
> I have energy in my hands and legs
>
> I get 'strong'
>
> I get bigger – raise my arms, stand up tall, move forward and use my hands to gesture
>
> I may physically engage – throwing, punching, smacking, kicking
>
> I find it hard to stop until the thing that threatens me is dealt with

Flight: I become avoidant

> I am unable to stay put as I want to get away from the thing threatening me
>
> I change the subject or use other distraction techniques
>
> I speak loudly/shout more, or my voice becomes quiet
>
> I have energy in my legs
>
> I get 'strong'

> I may physically disengage – moving slowly, walking or running away

> I find it hard to stop until the thing that threatens me is far enough away from me

My face gets red – a lot of blood got diverted to my eyes, ears, nose and brain

I get hot and start to sweat in preparation for the increase in body temperature that will come when I start running or fighting

I am focused on getting rid of the threat or away from it – nothing else

My sense of smell becomes more acute

I can sniff out stress-sweat others are giving off

I get a dry mouth

Producing saliva isn't important right now

My ability to sleep is minimal – it's not safe to. I find it hard to go to sleep. If I drift off, I don't sleep deeply in a way that restores me

My digestion is reduced and my appetite switches off

My immune system is reduced

My face may seem flat

My skin may seem paler (the blood has gone from under my skin to support my senses and muscles, and so I don't bleed too much if there is a fight and I get hurt superficially)

neocortex
not working

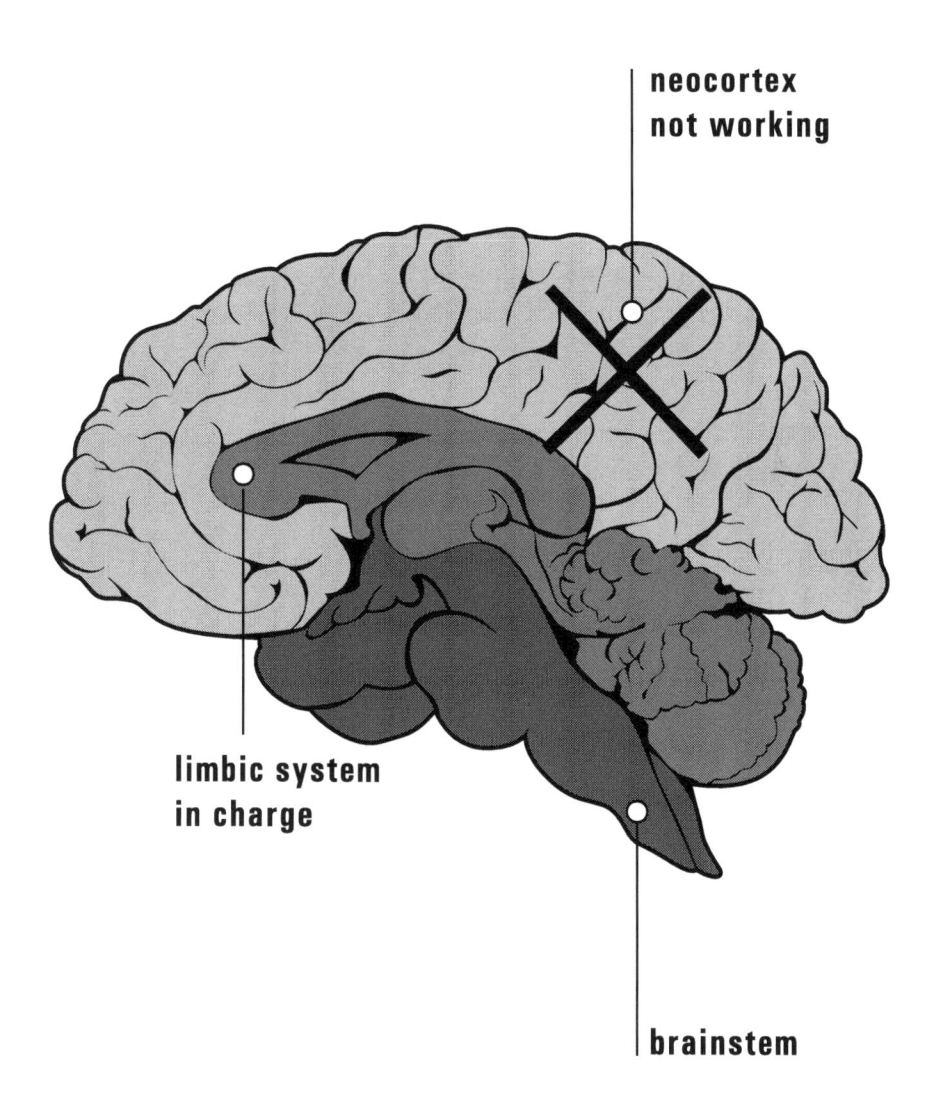

limbic system
in charge

brainstem

Fight/flight

Brain
My neocortex has gone 'offline'

I can no longer think well, plan or assess realistic outcomes. I cannot make good choices

I operate more from my limbic brain, where I have stored memories of experiences – things that happened to me matched with strong emotions. The memories get triggered and play out again, and it can sometimes feel like they are happening again

Interactions
I disengage from social interactions

I now read blank faces as angry/threatening

Unless you are clearly no threat to me (e.g. you are quiet, small, at a safe distance), I assume you are a danger

If other people move quickly around me I assume they are coming for me and I will respond to defend myself

If I'm not allowed to move (in an office or classroom), I will have to move in other ways – swinging on a chair, getting under a desk, wriggling, fiddling with things

Life view
I am *angry* about something ...

I feel invincible

or

I am *scared* right now ...

I feel vulnerable

or

I am worried or *anxious* about something in the future, or that I am thinking about ...

I feel vulnerable

I am not safe

I am not grounded

I am surviving

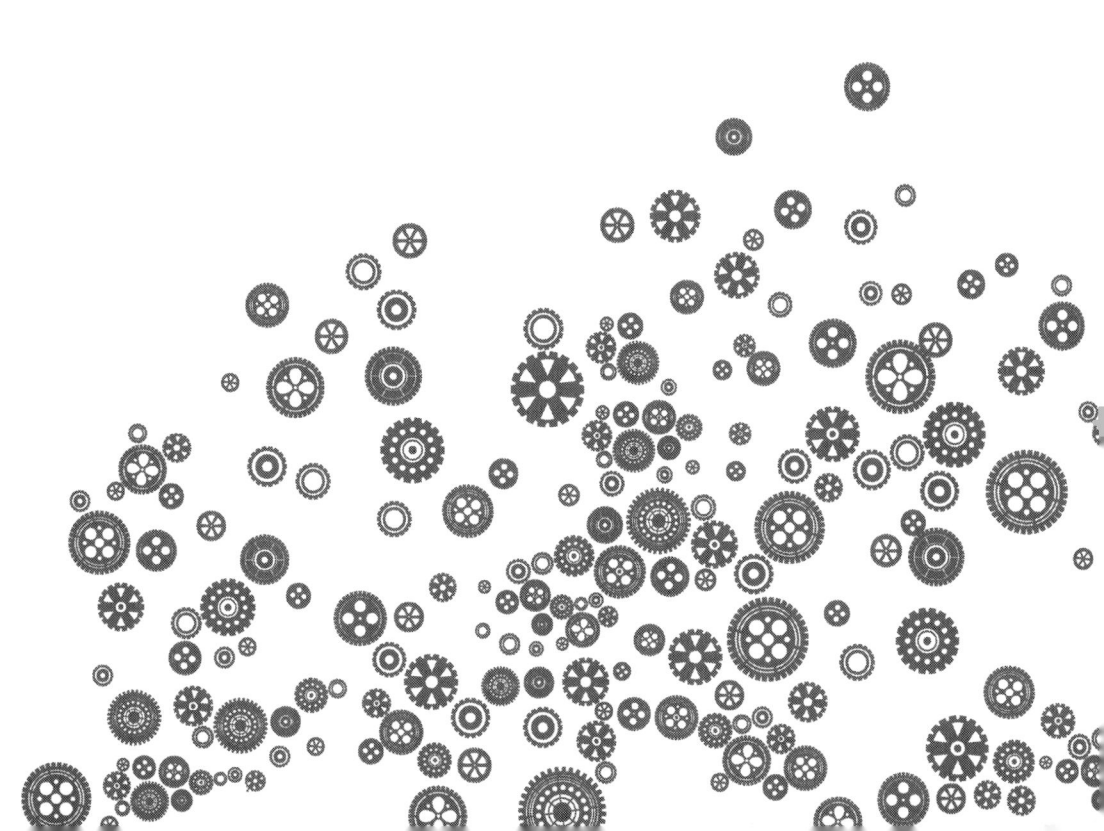

12

Immobilisation – Shut-down – Freeze

General state: My life is under threat

    Something very bad is happening

Nervous system: My sympathetic nervous system is shut down

I am operating from the oldest part of my brain, the brainstem – the bit I share with reptiles. My un-myelinated dorsal vagus nerve is the part of my nervous system functioning now. It works just to keep my basic functions working – heart rate, digestion, defecation and the sexual act

Eyes
I cannot make eye contact

Bright lights and quick movement are harder for me to cope with due to brain changes

Having too many things to process visually is overwhelming. I need empty space

Hearing
I cannot hear and understand

Body
My face is blank – no muscles moving

My digestion is shut off

My immune system is shut off

My appetite has gone

I can still go to the toilet – but may lose control over when

I become constipated or go to the toilet on the spot

My body is now also flooded with its own opioids – hormones to numb pain if/when the moment of death comes

I can't notice my body

I don't notice when I am hurt or there is pain

My muscles are very tight or very floppy

My heart rate is very high or very low

I find all of my body, or part of it, is stuck and hard to move

neocortex not working

limbic system not working

brainstem is keeping me alive

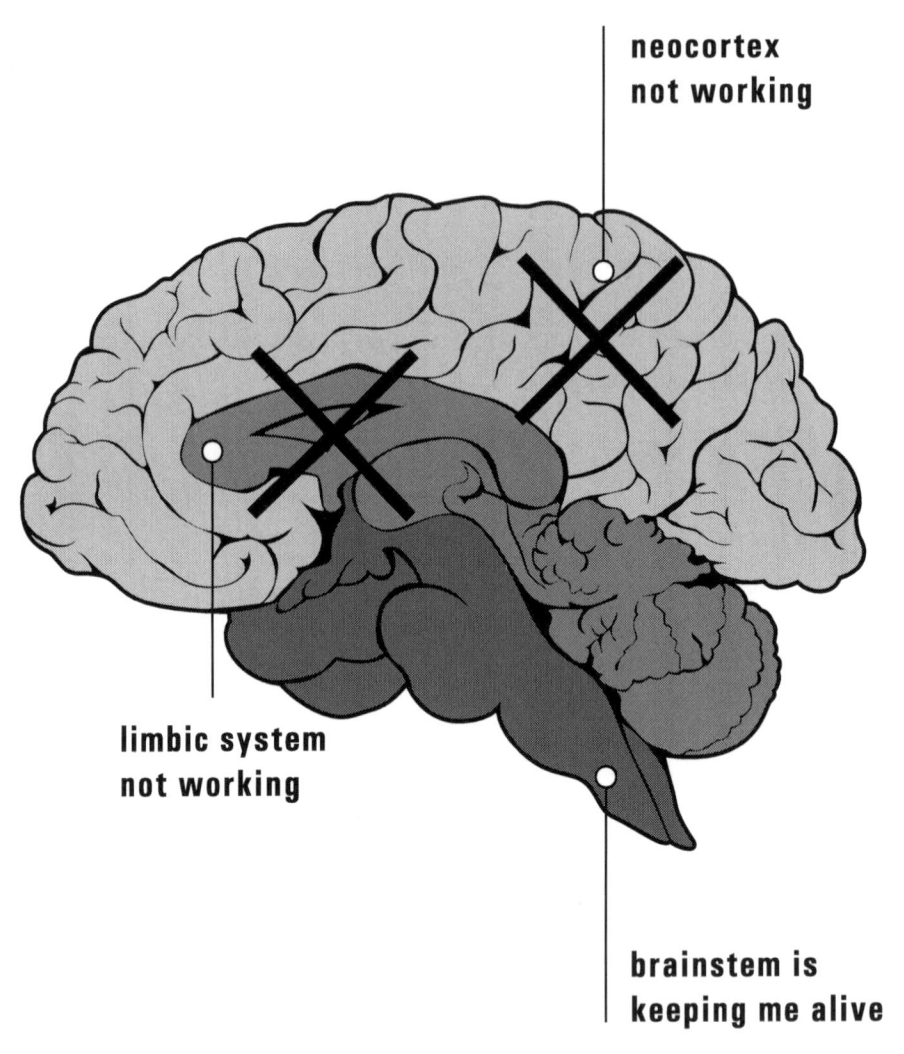

Freeze

Brain

My neocortex is offline, as is my limbic system. I am functioning mostly on my *reptilian brain*/brainstem

I find it almost impossible to speak, think, organise, plan or make choices

I am exclusively focused on surviving by not moving and by shutting down

I have no memory

I *dissociate*

My body is here but my 'head' isn't – this can actually feel really nice and floaty and calm

I know what's going on in my head – but have no connection with my body

I need to escape, but without moving

Interactions
I have no capacity for these and will certainly never initiate connections

I do not feel safe around people

I feel vulnerable

I try to isolate myself to feel safe

Functioning like this is incredibly hard – I just want to stay in my safe place (bed/home) all day

Life view
I am in 'freeze'

I am trying to save myself by becoming invisible

I cannot move forwards

I am stuck

I make myself small physically and in life. I don't want to be noticed

I am far from safe

I am nowhere near grounded

I am barely surviving

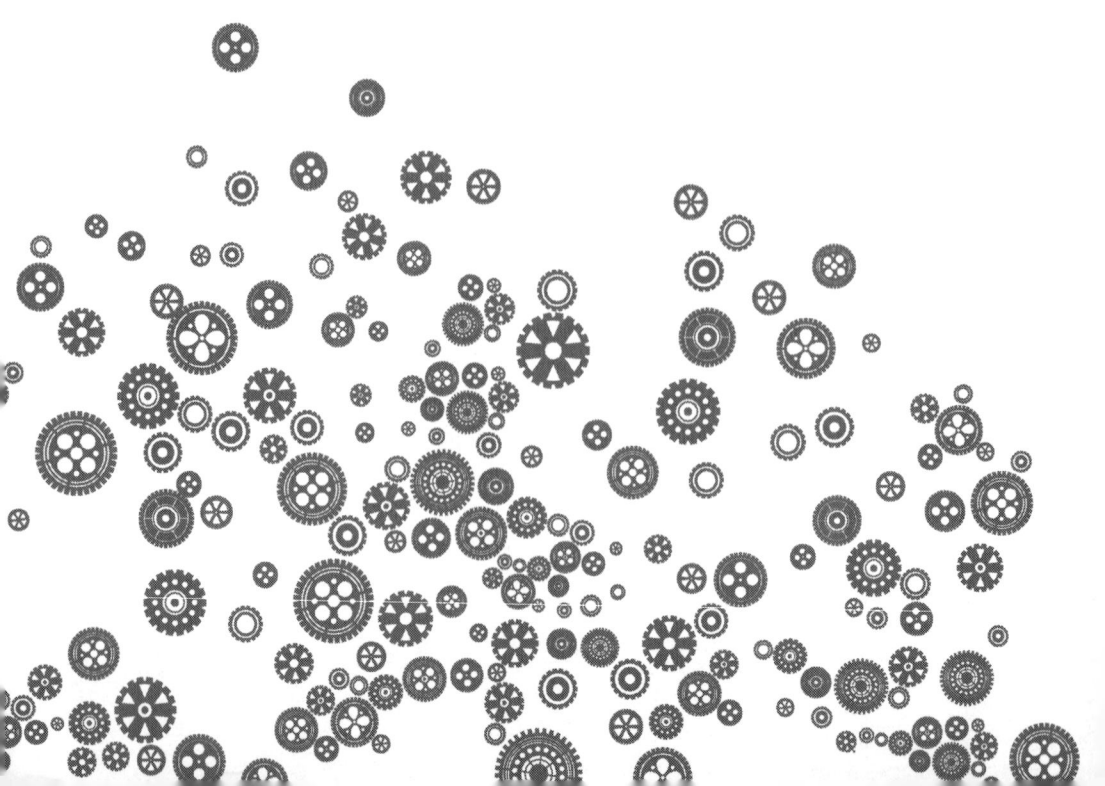

13

Taking It All In

I wouldn't be at all surprised if, as you read through the descriptions in the previous three chapters, you found yourself thinking about a particular child you know, work with or are related to ... or more than one.

It might be interesting to read through these lists again and think about yourself. These changes to our brain, our body and our subconscious outlook on life when we don't feel safe are the same whether we are five years old or sixty-five. If you really want to do some work and get more than you bargained for from this book, why not grab something to write with and journal through your answers to the following questions?

- When do you notice yourself operating in the different states?
- Do you identify with one of these states more than others?
- When you feel unsafe, do you go into mobilisation via 'fight' or 'flight', or do you instantly shut down?
- Do you use different approaches in different situations (work, home, friends, extended family)?
- What is a childhood memory of not feeling safe – and which state did you go into?

If you identify times when you function in each of the survival states, it might be helpful to read through that list a final time, and consider what changes those around you see or experience in you when you are in that state.

14

Can't Decide! (Functional Freeze)

Did you go back through those lists? Did you struggle to identify with just one ... because you actually identify with two?

If you recognise elements of the 'Freeze' state in how you live in the world (feeling distant, disconnected from life or others, struggling to find joy or experience deep peace, or trying to do your best while also staying invisible), but also recognise the huge energy of the 'Mobilisation' states on your inside, then you may be feeling a bit confused round about now. Please do not worry. This is really common, so let's explore it. If you don't relate to this, then you can skip to the next chapter – or stick with me to understand what life is like for many others.

The Freeze state, when it is full-blown freeze, leads the body to total shut-down. People literally find it next to impossible to move arms or legs, stand up, sit down etc. There is no way there will be any eye contact, or anything other than a flat facial expression. There will be no sound, no speech, no signs of life. So does this mean that, if someone is not totally frozen to the spot and unable to move, they are not really in a state of Freeze?

No.

When people get overwhelmed, often as little children, by something horrible that they cannot fight or get away from, their system will shut down internally and their body will hold the patterns of tension in muscles as well as the stored energy that they would have used to fight or run if they could have done so. That huge internal energy often doesn't just dissipate on its own, and can stay in the body for years, or even decades. The trapped energy from the adrenaline and cortisol hormones will now be used to 'drive' that person to keep functioning in life.

It is not at all unusual for brilliant people who seem to have achieved so much in their 20s, 30s and 40s to express a sense of being distant from their own life or disconnected from others, or find it hard to feel joy, pleasure, peace or deep satisfaction. Yet these same people seem to have been set on 'go' for as long as they can remember – 'it's just who I am'. They may burn up hours in the gym or socialising after long days at work. They may feel a deep need to keep going, to keep pushing on and not stop. They may find relaxing, sleeping in, and sitting 'doing nothing' harder than getting more degrees or qualifications. They hardly notice their body – they needed to dissociate from the pain of what happened to them and their body when they were little. They just live in their heads … and keep pushing on as long as their overwhelmed body can.

This is the *Functional Freeze* – a term coined by Peter Levine, whose background is in medical biophysics and psychology. He is another incredible contributor to our understanding of nervous systems.

If you can relate to the metaphor that life feels like you are driving along with one foot flat on the accelerator and the other pressing hard on the brake pedal, then it may well be that your body, your nervous system, is in Functional Freeze.

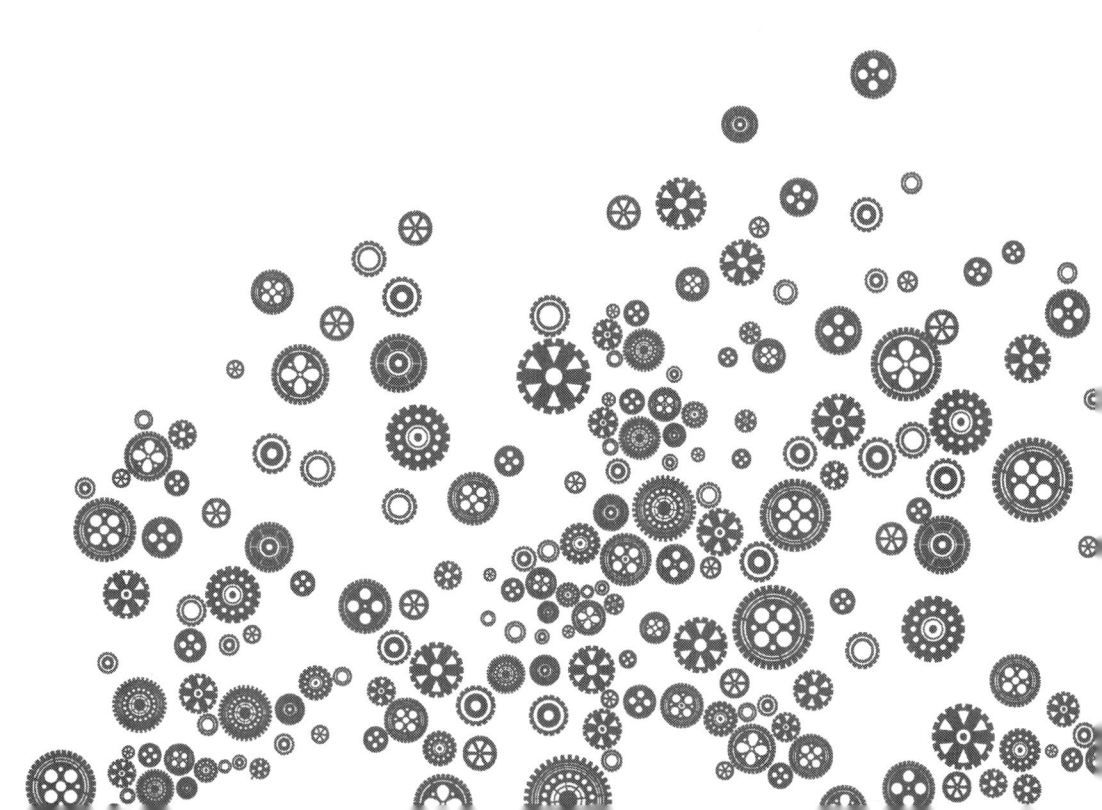

15

Hearing

Did you notice how one of the things that happens when someone doesn't feel safe is that their hearing changes?

Wonky hearing
Several years ago, I was in a road traffic accident. It was a bit dramatic in that it resulted in closure of the M25 motorway on a Friday evening in rush hour but, miraculously, no one was physically harmed. I had whiplash, but nothing was physically broken, which was quite amazing, considering that my car was a write-off, having been hit by a lorry. I will never forget how, after being checked over by paramedics at the side of the motorway, they dropped me off at a nearby pub. I waited there for a taxi to pick me up to take me to my destination.

It was as I was sitting in the pub, still trying to get my head around what had happened, that I realised my hearing was wonky. I could hear the music playing in the background *so* loudly – I couldn't believe it wasn't bothering anybody else there! When the landlord came to see if he could get me a drink (non-alcoholic!), I could barely hear him. I was overwhelmed by the sounds from the background and couldn't hear the guy standing right by me.

I didn't understand it then, but that was one of the elements of the change in my physiology from the traumatic experience. I had clung on to my steering wheel and gone into freeze, with all that meant for my brain and body functions. I totally understand how hard it is for children who have experienced trauma and find themselves in a classroom trying to sift out the teacher's voice or to hear what the dinner lady is saying to them. I can also understand those children struggling to hear and understand one voice speaking to them in a classroom if they don't feel fully safe for some reason, and those out with parents in a shopping centre, pub, soft-play park or other noisy setting. It makes sense. These children are not being naughty, evasive or rude. They genuinely can't hear properly. It is not likely that their hearing needs support, but rather that their nervous system needs help to find safety again. As my nervous system found its way back to grounded (with some professional help and over a period of time), my hearing got back to normal again.

Sounds of safety
The way our ears change when we don't feel safe is really interesting when we think about children, and especially their speech development. The changes in the middle ear happen when we need to go into a defensive state, and – like the mummy bear I mentioned earlier – we check out our environment and use our senses to search for information as to where the danger is lurking. In normal everyday life, even though children don't need to scan their surroundings for wolves or any other predator, if they are not grounded, they will still be on alert trying to detect danger. The animal world knows that the sounds of threat are generally in the low frequencies – the growls and roars of animals before they attack. That is what middle ears attune to: lower frequencies and sounds of danger.

It is interesting to understand this for the children who struggle with male teachers who have a naturally deep voice, or those who were fine at home with Mum but become distressed when they hear Dad coming home. If there is no other reason a child would be afraid of their dad, then this is worth considering. The simple fact of the lower register of Dad's deeper voice can be interpreted in their activated nervous system as sounds of threat.

Children often miss hearing the ends of words when their hearing is compromised, as mine was, due to being in a threatened state. If they are babies in overwhelm, freeze or shut-down, their hearing development can be significantly halted, which obviously also affects their speech. Attempts to focus only on repairing speech difficulties without addressing the nervous system may well have limited benefit or take a lot of work for little gain.

Safe to talk

Ben was a gorgeous little guy who I had the privilege of working with. He had experienced physical abuse at the hands of his dad from the age of six months. It was several years later when I met him in pre-school; he was away from danger now, living safely with his devoted mum. However, he was still in freeze. His speech was severely delayed and, although most of my play therapy clients who experienced trauma in early life started sessions with speech difficulties, his was the most severe I had ever come across.

Ben's nervous system was still in a state of overwhelmed shut-down. The environment of his classroom was also pretty overwhelming for him. The moving bodies, the noise of the talking, singing, shouting, the toys and the inevitable crying were all too much for him to process in his freeze state. One of the big concerns the school had was his speech, and conscientiously they had already referred him to speech and language sessions. They weren't getting anywhere. As I started to work with Ben I asked that those sessions be put on hold so he wasn't getting too many differing approaches at the same time, which is always tricky for a child. The school and the speech therapist were happy to oblige – there were plenty more children on the waiting list!

I was highly mindful of myself every time I arrived at the school for his play therapy session. I would sit in my car and check in with my body – notice what was going on in me and how grounded I was. Just getting into the school often brought interaction with stressed adults, and setting up the room for our sessions often involved navigating surprises of things 'missing'. After I got our room ready, and before I collected Ben, I would check in with my body again, and use my own grounding toolkit to get myself and my nervous system safe for his. A few months later, Ben was 'melting', as his mum put it, describing how she knew he was coming out of his 'freeze' and coming back to life.

A few months after that, without having had any focus on his speech at all, Ben was chatting happily and starting to catch up with his peers. His body was no longer stuck in freeze, and that changed his neurophysiology, including his middle ear – he heard more of what was going on around him and, because his neocortex had come back online and was functioning for him again, he was able to process those sounds more effectively and started to move his mouth to recreate the sounds and words himself.

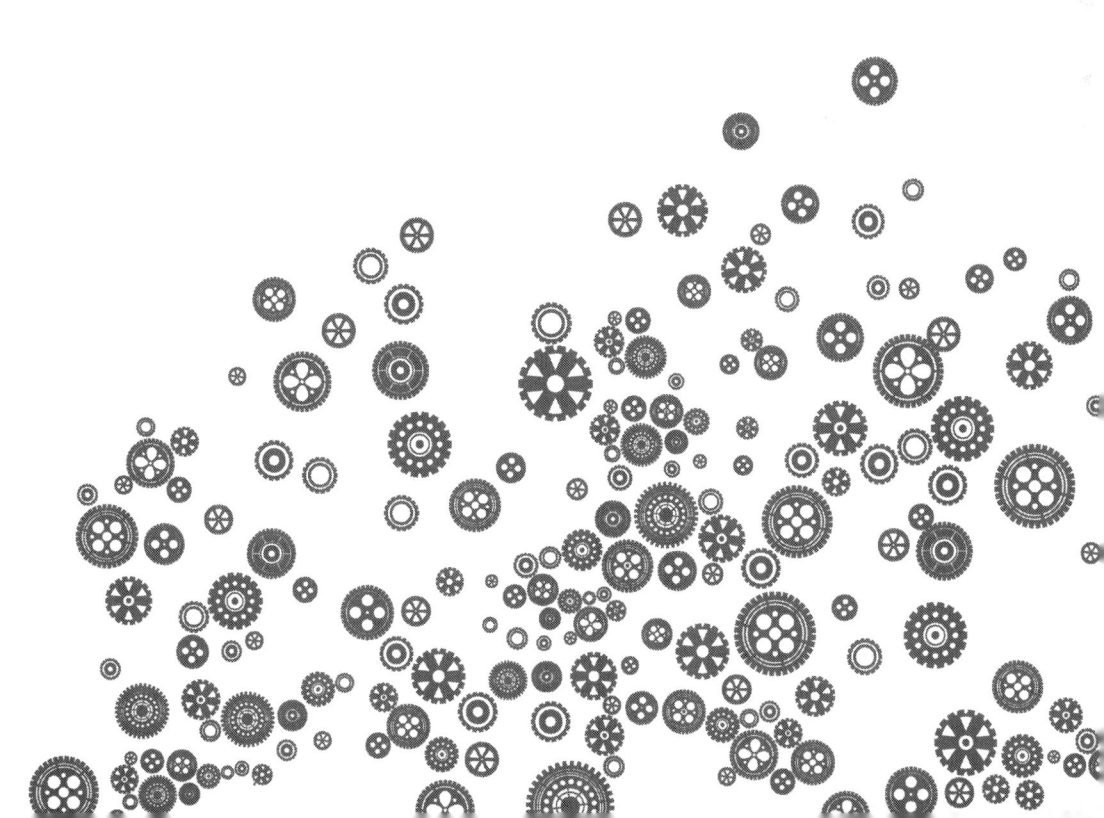

16

It Is Not A Conscious Choice

However much we may wish it to be different, we need to appreciate that the changes that go on in a child's brain and body when they do not feel safe, or feel that things are dangerous or that their life is under threat, are *not* under their conscious control.

For example, if they do not feel safe, they *cannot make the 'thinking part' of their brain – the prefrontal cortex – work*. It has gone offline, however many times we encourage them to 'make a good choice'.

If they feel under threat, they may well be *unable to hear and process* what we are saying, even if we think we spoke clearly enough.

If they feel totally overwhelmed and they have gone into freeze, they will *never be able to give you eye contact*, no matter how many times you say, "look at me when I'm talking to you".

Of course, there are times when a child is still feeling safe(ish) and is testing out their boundaries, trying to make a point and wilfully ignoring us. As the grown-ups, we need to be able to tune in and know the difference. When a child is not feeling safe, their nervous system reacts, and their brain, body and behaviour respond; they don't *choose* to be difficult, confrontational, non-responsive, avoidant or unable to concentrate etc.

If we as adults can understand these unconscious changes, we can practise noticing when we are not grounded. From this place of noticing ourselves better first, we can focus on becoming proficient at noticing the changes that happen in the children around us. We can also consider, with honesty, what may have triggered them to being in this 'not safe' state, and in this way we can give these children the incredible gift of being understood.

The Jenny conundrum

Jenny was not understood. She was a conundrum. The adults around her were confused about what was going on with her.

Jenny was struggling – that much was clear. However, no one could understand why this was. Last year, she had been fine – or, at least, significantly more 'fine' than now: she had responded to her teacher, she was calmer, she even wrote – and wrote well.

Now she was all over the place: constantly moving her body; pushing boundaries, getting into altercations with children in her class; spending time isolating herself – in the toilets, on the classroom windowsill or under her desk. She hardly made eye contact with anyone and barely ever risked putting pen to paper.

Her parents loved their daughter.

Jenny's mum was anxious. She cared a lot and worried a lot, and was doing her absolute best for her daughter. Her muscles were tight, her energy low, she held a lot of emotion and a lot of tension in her body, and she frequently felt on the verge of tears.

Jenny's dad was passionate – a man of action. He cared a lot, had strong energy and a quick temper, and wanted to get things fixed. He worked hard, was tired as a result and had held in a lot of emotion through the years – even from before Jenny was born. He loved his little girl to bits, but his frustration at not understanding her and not being able to control her behaviour was adding to his money worries and getting the better of him more and more.

Jenny's teacher was emotionally frozen. She was there in body and walked through the required routine every day, for as long as she could take. She was putting up a brave 'everything's fine' front, but inside she was struggling. This new job was just so hard for her – she spent a lot of time feeling out of her depth. It was a familiar feeling that haunted her and made her feel as if she would get found out – be exposed – at any minute. This made her feel like running away. She hid it well, though, and she stayed. She physically stuck it out as long as she could, but emotionally had disconnected from the class, the school and the whole job. When children were struggling, she had nothing to resource them with but threats, consequences and the school rules. Her voice was shrill. She was tense and edgy; people couldn't get near. She snapped and shouted, often not making sense, being rational or fair. She turned a blind eye to much of what went on in her junior class – until something happened that warranted sending the 'offenders' out of her room, away from her. She wanted them away – distance was her survival tool.

There was one teacher to whom Jenny consistently responded well. Miss Timms was one person she was able to really hear, understand and respond to as her best self. Everyone marvelled at this and wondered why. Some were jealous, others mystified. It was a conundrum. Why was it that Jenny would do whatever she was asked or told by her but there was likely to be a drama with the others?

Jenny was a bright girl – she knew she was a 'problem'. She knew people had meetings about her. She knew she needed help – and that everyone wanted to help her. She knew that because she had lost count of the times they told her. Her head knew it. Her head got the message. But her body just didn't believe.

Mystery unravelled

Jenny's body reacted to the bodies around her. She detected instantly whether they were grounded, calm and safe, or not safe themselves and therefore also unsafe, and threatening to her. Her subconscious radar was acutely attuned and detected the threat levels coming from the bodies – the nervous systems – the muscles and energy around her.

One person beeped on her threat-detection radar as *unstable: flight patterns*. Take survival action.

One was indicating *unstable: aggressive – fight*. Take survival action.

One indicated as *very unstable: absent – frozen* – shut down for most of the time – but occasionally also *fight*. Take significant survival action.

One, however, registered *grounded*. *Calm*, body position never threatened. Gentle, sing-song voice, with a slightly higher pitch when speaking to her. Words that indicated she understood. Genuine smiles. When their eyes met (and they did), it was *safe*.

When this lady spoke, Jenny's body still felt OK. She could still think, understand, reason and be curious and creative. When Miss Timms asked her to do something, Jenny did it. She heard what this lady said, more than other people, so it was easier to follow through, simply because she had heard properly. Miss Timms kept her feeling calm – or, if she was angry or upset, Miss Timms could help her get calm.

Everyone cared about Jenny. Everyone wanted to help her, but none of the other key adults understood how hard they made it for her in the way they spoke, the way their faces looked, the way their muscles were tight, the way their voices sounded, the way they moved and the tension they held. The way they were.

Everyone wanted the best for her, but there was only one person Jenny knew was a consistent resource to really help her – both mind and body. When she was around this lady, things were easier, calmer and more straightforward. Being with her made Jenny feel OK, present, alive – safer.

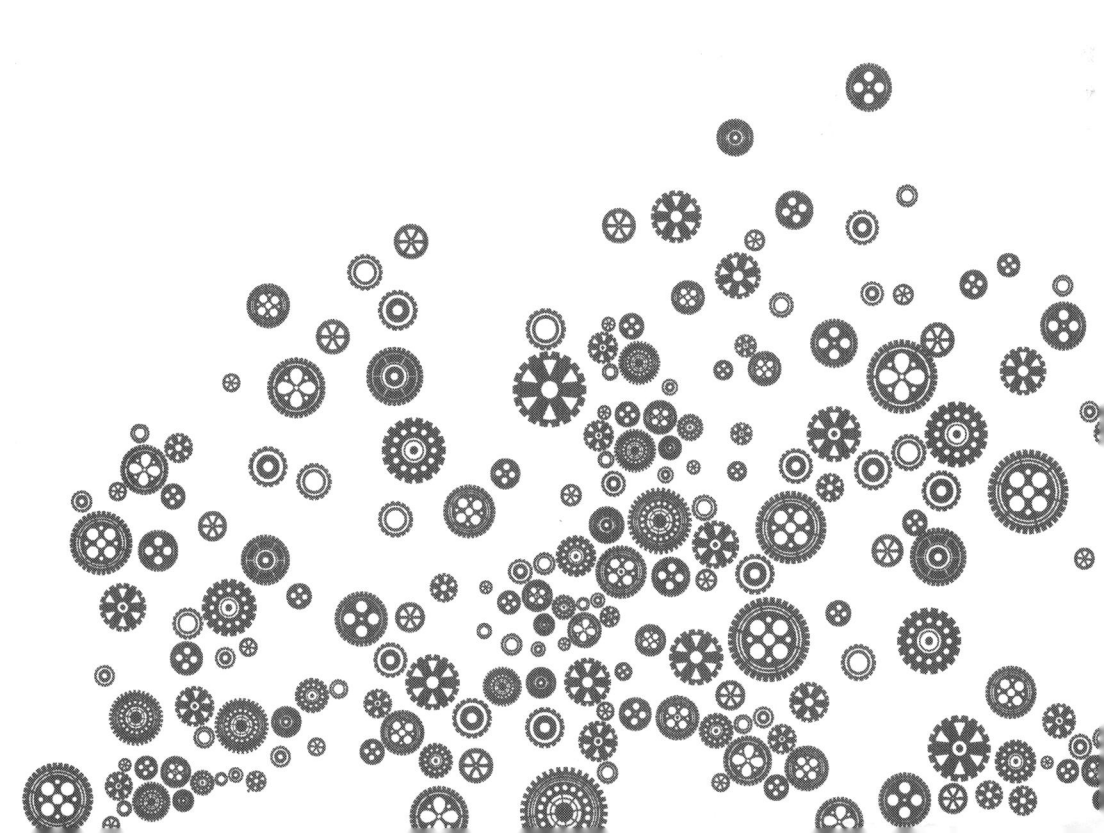

17

Don't Waste Your Time

Dr Bruce Perry is another legend in the world of understanding children, brains and how to bring out the best in the children around us. He is a psychiatrist who continues to research into how the brain develops and how relationships affect us as we grow. One of the key points he makes in his training is relevant for us here.

He says that, if we are with a child whose nervous system is dysregulated – which is another way of saying highly activated, because they don't feel safe – then their brain won't be functioning fully. We already know this from the descriptions of what happens to our 'thinking brain' (neocortex) in the chapters on Mobilisation (Chapter 11) and Immobilisation (12). Dr Perry goes on to say (not quite in these words) that if we think we can talk to, reason with and get any sense from a child while their 'thinking' brain is offline, we are deluding ourselves. Any time we spend trying to get children to think, explain themselves or perform in any way while they are feeling extremely unsafe is time wasted.

Having spent many hours with children who know what it is like to have experienced these states of 'dysregulation', I think it is important to take this one step further. These children have told me about being aware that their teacher or parent is talking to them, wanting an answer from them. They have explained how they have been confused: how come they just could not think about or understand what was being said, or provide what the adult wanted? If they could have given the right answer, or any answer, they would have done so. It would have been the quickest, surest way to make the adult happy and make this moment stop.

Freezing into homework

James is one example. A really popular boy in his class, he was often one of the first picked when it was time to choose teams in PE. He could move well and was a great encourager of others, too. When he was outside he felt alive, free and as if he could keep up and match his peers. In the classroom, however, it was a different story. He struggled to read and found his eyes darting about all over the page, unable to focus on the words in front of him. When his teacher was having a 'bad day' and was more shouty than usual, this seemed to make things worse for James. Often, words on a page would blur, but if he concentrated really hard, made a slight smile on his face and blinked just the right way, he could sometimes get them to come back again. He was great in class discussions and was happy to put his hand up to share what his brilliant brain thought. It was just when it was time for the reading or writing that he struggled – always struggling most on the teacher's 'bad days'.

One evening at home, although his mum was really busy, she made time to do his homework with him before bath-time. Although she hadn't said anything, he could just tell that she was not OK; she was cranky and loud and rushing. With the dirty plates still piled up on the side, they sat down at the kitchen table and he knew he wanted to get through this as fast as he could, so she could get on with the other jobs on her list. In all honesty, he wished he could have done his homework alone. He didn't really want to be sitting here with her when she had other things she needed to get to. He felt her pressure.

Already the pressure in his body was growing. He was starting to feel his stomach tighten and the heat come into his cheeks. She asked him to tell her what he had to do for homework. He couldn't remember. She asked again, with a little 'weren't you listening to your teacher?' comment thrown in. Yes, he had been listening, but right now his brain was feeling fuzzy and he couldn't find that answer for her. His mum pulled the work out of his book bag and put it on the table in front of him, slightly slapping it down on the table, and pushing it in front of him with a force that let him know she was getting more annoyed. He started to feel sick. The room started to close in and he realised he was sitting in the corner. His mum was blocking his exit. He felt trapped.

Over the next few minutes, James became hotter, crosser and tighter – and then it went quiet. He was still seated at the table, but he stopped fiddling with his pencil. He stopped being able to hear what she was saying to him. He was just staring. His mum thought he was being rude and 'blanking her' on purpose. She didn't appreciate his behaviour as she was the one giving up her time to sit with him when she had lots of other things she could be doing. After ten minutes there was still no sign of homework actually getting done. Each passing minute was heaping more shame into his self-worth; more proof that he was rubbish; more evidence that he was a failure.

This is a scenario I have seen play out and have heard about from so many confused children that I know there are many children like James going through this at home and/or at school. When a child is not functioning in their 'social engagement' physiology, they will move to explore the fight/flight options. If those are not realistic options to make this threatening situation go away – because the child is physically not able to get out past the adult, or maybe because they are aware they cannot shout or express any angry energy around or *at* their teacher or parent – they will shut down. As James's situation so graphically describes, when children are not feeling safe, we are not only wasting time trying to reason with them, trying to get them to think or to explain themselves, but the longer we keep pressure on them to perform while they are shut down, the more impact it can have on their self-esteem.

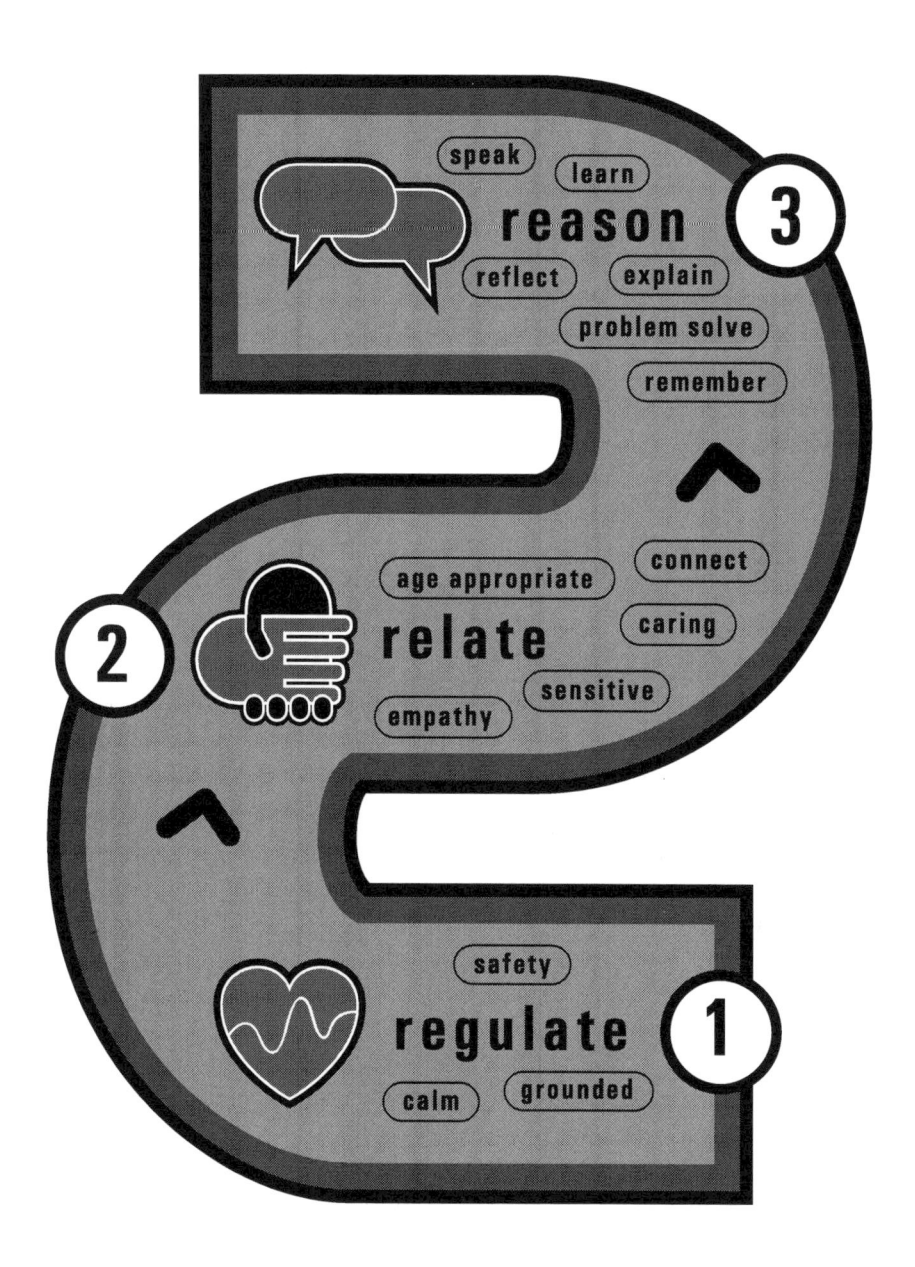

3 reason
speak, learn, reflect, explain, problem solve, remember

2 relate
age appropriate, connect, caring, sensitive, empathy

1 regulate
safety, calm, grounded

Adapted, with permission, from © Bruce D. Perry

Dr Perry describes three stages: Regulate. Relate. Reason. For bringing the best out of any child, we need to be supporting them in that order.

1. Helping to *regulate* their nervous system – i.e. helping them become calm and access their social engagement set-up – is the absolute first and fundamental priority. This will slow breathing, regulate heart rate, and allow their brainstem to establish a sense of 'safety' for the body.

2. From here we then need to *relate* to the child, to reconnect with them in a way that reminds them we are safe and there for them.

3. Only when the child is regulated and feeling OK with the connection they have with us can we finally begin to explore the *reasons* around what is going on. Reasoning is governed by the cortex – the thinking brain. If this is not online, because the child's nervous system is still dysregulated, we waste our time – and theirs. Sadly, this is what happens every time a child is required to 'explain what happened' while they are still hot and angry from the skirmish on the playground. It is what happens when an anxious child in pre-panic-attack mode is asked to explain exactly what they are scared of. It is what happens when we want children to do something, say something or explain something and they are more focused on simply feeling safe again.

When we understand the way the brain and body function when under pressure, in danger or under threat, the wisdom in these stages is obvious. However, breaking the habit of going straight to the 'reason' bit when trying to 'help' a child can take some time. Building a new habit of walking these '3Rs' in order will take time and intention to develop. One thing is clear, though: there is no point in even *trying* to help regulate, relate or reason with a child if our own nervous system is not grounded.

SECTION 3

GROUNDED

Children are educated by what
the grown-up is and not by his talk.

Carl Jung

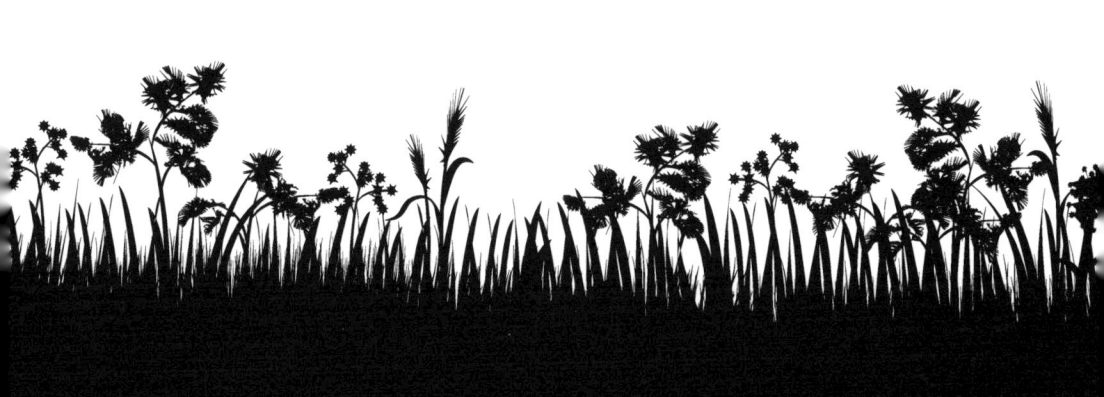

18

Surviving When You Need To Survive

There is a time and a place for everything.

When we need to deal with a real threat, we must get on and deal with it. If there is genuine physical or emotional danger, then bringing out our best – for us and a child – means using those amazing survival states that we were made with. The best 'us' in an emergency obviously requires us to make use of our mobilisation resources. When there is a genuine threat to physical safety for yourself or a child, go right on into your best-chance God-given surviving state and do what needs to be done. Get away from danger or challenge it to make it no longer a threat. It's OK to do what it takes to get you and the child safe again.

Please do not feel bad if you remember shouting, being aggressive, or moving a child away from a dangerous situation or people, *if* there was a genuine threat and you acted to keep yourself and that child physically safe. The child may well have been scared by what happened – but at least you will be able to take whatever time they need to process it all, if you are both still alive and when you are safe again. If they were scared by what happened, by you shouting or pulling them or pushing them away from something, there will be time afterwards to talk them back through it and hear their experiences. They will need to be able to say what it was like for them. They will need to be really heard. After listening to their side of the story, you can apologise if they were scared by something you did and reassure them that you were acting to keep them safe.

Our mobilisation response is there for a reason, just like our freeze response. When the time is right, we need them to survive. However, they are generally not necessary for our normal day-to-day lives, and we do best, we thrive, when we are grounded.

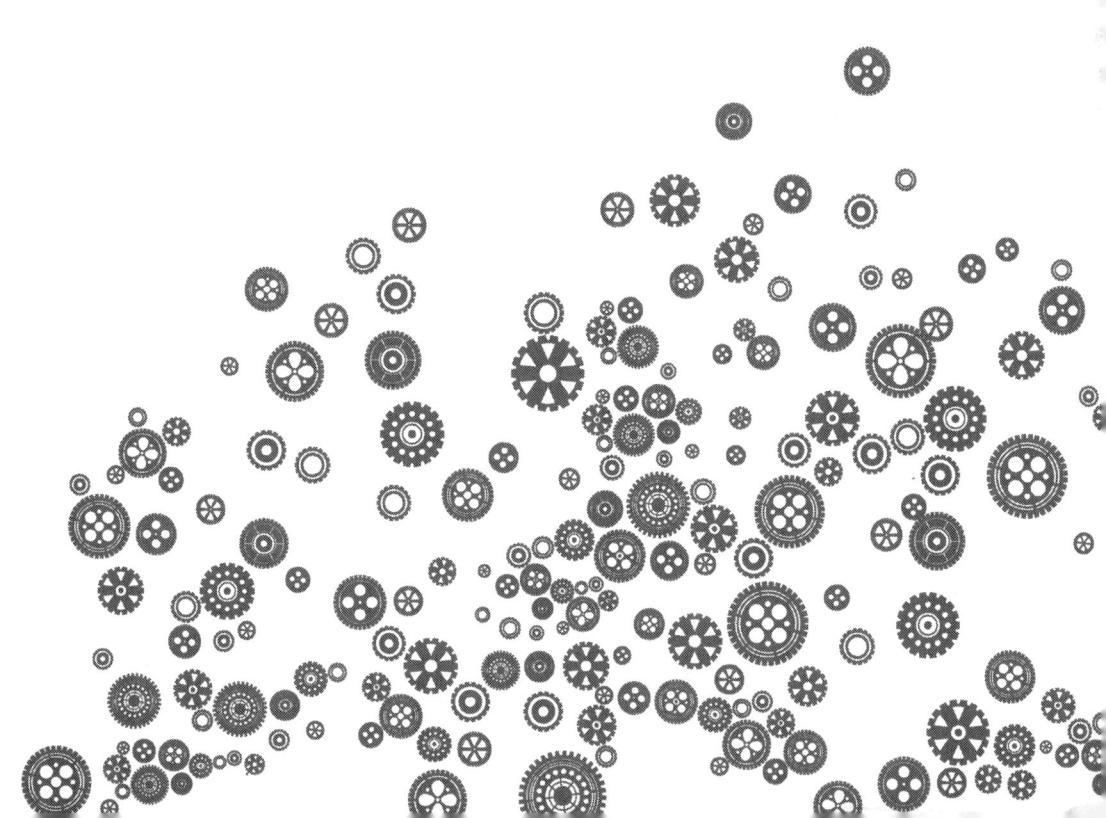

19

What Is Grounded?

We now realise that, whether we are angry, stressed, anxious, fearful, overwhelmed or in emotional shut-down and not feeling anything right now, the state our body is in sends a message to the children around us. Bodies communicate. The children subconsciously know we are not OK and things are not OK – and therefore, potentially, *they* are not OK, either ... and their survival make-myself-safe behaviours begin. The only way we can guarantee that we can bring out the best in us – and be the best, safe, approachable resource for them – is if we are grounded. In other words: if we can bring the level of activation in our nervous system down to the point where we leave behind our defensive (mobilisation) behaviours and operate in our social engagement physiology.

Grounded can do

When we are grounded, we can:

- Use all our thinking, problem-solving, rational brain
- Be empathetic and see someone else's point of view
- Keep a genuine smile on our face: cheeks, mouth and eyes
- Speak calmly and clearly, without a 'tone'
- Be able to cope with someone else's emotions, without taking their upset personally (unless we should!)
- Really listen and objectively, want to understand their experience or point of view
- Be calm and still in our body
- Smell nice (!), i.e. no unconscious fear pheromones
- Bring a calm, assertive air of 'I am in control of myself/this classroom/this situation'

- Think about how best to defuse a situation or help the other person become more grounded/calm themselves (and saying 'calm down' is never the way to go!)

Grounded

If you search for a definition of this word, you will find many. Like 'traumatic', it has wheedled its way into our modern vocabulary and is often used in ways that are not completely accurate in scientific terms.

People often say 'grounded' when they mean simply 'calmer' or 'better'. For example: "I went for a walk in the park and felt more grounded"; "listening to music helps me get grounded"; or "breathing exercises are a way I can ground myself".

There are two definitions that I particularly like.

The first is from David Berceli, an international expert in working with traumatised people, who describes 'grounded' as:

> ... in full awareness and connection with
> What's going on inside me,
> What's going on in my environment
> And what's going on with other people near me.

The second is by Bessel van der Kolk, a legend in the current field of healing trauma, who says:

> 'Grounded' means that you can feel your butt in your chair, see the light coming through the window, feel the tension in your calves, and hear the wind stirring in the tree outside.

Sounds lovely, doesn't it? It is actually harder than it first seems. Many of us have become proficient at noticing what's going on around us and what's going on with other people, and yet we are *unaware of ourselves and the internal experience of our body*.

Conversely, we may be so absorbed with every nuance of change within ourselves that we are not connected with those around us, or even notice what is going on in our environment.

However much we want it and can understand the benefits to those around us, it *takes real practice to become proficient at being grounded* and sustaining that state for any period of time.

Incidentally, being grounded *permanently* is highly unlikely. If you think you are, or know someone who says they are because they've done a million hours of meditation etc., it is entirely possible that they are dissociated. This is another element of our body's survival tool kit and involves flooding our system with opioids. Not surprisingly, then, it can feel quite nice, calm and floaty! Similar to the 'shut-down/freeze' state, it doesn't have any real awareness of or connection with the body. It might feel very 'zen', but if you still can't notice and describe your internal body sensations, it is unlikely that you are grounded, and children may subconsciously detect you as 'not really fully there' = 'not able to keep us safe'.

It is normal and natural that we will at certain times (some more than others) be ungrounded. As a life skill, to be able to really notice when we are not grounded and to know what to do to help ourselves move into that state would be top of my list for life-skills education! In fact, I am so convinced of this that I am working on exactly this with the staff and children of a local primary school.

Before we get into ways to become more grounded, let's take a look at the challenges we are up against.

20

What Stops Us Being The Calm, Grounded Adults We Want To Be?

Another way of asking the same question is: "What kinds of things will change our nervous system away from our 'social engagement' safe protocol and move us into one of our survival states?".

The answer is: almost anything!

All sorts of everyday events can mean our nervous system shifts us away from feeling safe and being grounded. Here are just a few examples.

Everyday events
Deadlines – a man-made threat

Being somewhere on time when you are running late

Trying to keep up appearances

Being observed at work or at home

Being put on the spot or having to explain yourself

Exams, tests, assessments

Being shouted at

Hearing someone shouting/screaming at someone else

Losing something important (money, keys, phone, pet)

Hearing loud noises that you weren't expecting

House alarms, car alarms, fire alarms

Rushing to cram more into our days than we can comfortably fit in

Interacting with people who are upset, angry, anxious or depressed

Other people's bad driving

Going somewhere that feels unsafe

Being with unpredictable people (children or adults)

Public speaking

Watching something upsetting

Feeling manipulated or taken for granted

Low blood-sugar levels

Inadequate or unrestful sleep

Someone looking away from you or turning their back

Meetings, appointments, interviews

Being responsible for others in any way

Managing emergencies, big or small

Being in unsafe situations with someone else

Being criticised

Being hurt by an animal

Accidents or injuries

Medical procedures – screening, scans, injections

The dentist's chair

Clearly none of these are genuinely life-endangering situations! However, the more stress and tension our bodies harbour, the more quickly we will react significantly to other blips, challenges or life's twists and turns.

It's not just about now
Did you know that, however much we try and live in the present and focus on being driven by our highly active 'heads', our bodies still hold the tension patterns of past experiences? It is entirely possible that a nervous system put into a significant state of fight, flight or freeze in years gone by can still be functioning from that place. It may feel like 'normal' because it is familiar, but others will probably notice and children, especially, can still detect the activation and feel unsafe around us.

Experiences that may still be lingering in your body tension and your nervous system may include:

Past traumatic experiences

Birth trauma

Developmental trauma

Being raised in an unpredictable or unsafe atmosphere at home due to siblings or parents/carers

Being raised in a dangerous location

Accidents or injuries

Illnesses, hospital stays, operations

Abuse (physical, emotional, sexual or neglect)

Mass terrifying events: terrorist attacks, war, fires, bombings, shootings etc.

Long-term stress situations, at home or at work

Long-term caring for another (adult or child)

If we are living and doing our best in the present every day following a life story that includes *any* experience on the list above, we may find that our desire for re-regulating our nervous system and establishing our own 'grounded-ness' will take more work for us than for someone who has not experienced any major incidents that have impacted their nervous system. The good news is that it is entirely possible to get there, and I have worked with many parents and professionals over the years who would tell you this. However, making that journey is a choice, and will only happen by choice, intention and decision, not by magic. Sometimes, though, 'life' encourages us by holding up a mirror to help us see more clearly who we are at a moment in time.

Breakfast to lunchtime via the school gate and classrooms

Susan had been worried about her financial situation for a while. For various reasons, things were looking bleak. She was finally free of the abusive partner she had spent the previous ten years submitting to and appeasing in every possible way to keep her and her teenage daughter safe from his raging, but it meant she was now on her own, having to make ends meet.

She hadn't slept well, and had had an epic argument with her daughter just before they left for school. She dropped her daughter off after a journey that was geographically short but felt so very long. The sound of the car door slamming broke the stony silence, and Susan continued to the school where she worked. She had brushed off the 'are you OK'? enquiries while she put her bags away, and was still seething and as tight as concrete in her stomach when she got outside for gate-duty. Today was her day to be there to talk to parents and welcome children in with a smile – which she knew might require a bit of forced matter-of-professional-choice this morning.

There were often one or two parents who would use this time to vent their frustrations, concerns and anxieties on whichever member of staff was on the gate. That was normal and to be expected. But five? Five different parents choosing that day to get into verbal fisticuffs with her – really?

The bell rang, and she sought sanctuary in the school building, taking time to grab a quick drink before she was due in class. Covering two different classes that morning meant that she had interactions, in close proximity, with a further 60 children. By lunchtime, several children from both classes – interestingly, the ones who were well known for struggling with their behaviour at the best of times – were all congregated outside the Head's office.

Was it all coincidence?

Maybe.

Sitting in a training course in the afternoon, Susan was learning about how we subconsciously read others and pick up on their stress. If they are not safe, we notice and we have to work hard to keep ourselves grounded. More often than not, though – especially if we are children – we just react. The morning ran back through her mind at high speed. She could feel the worry she woke up with, and how quickly that had escalated into the angry energy she had carried in her body … and on her face … and in her tone of voice. She realised that she was the constant. She was the one 'at the scene' of each difficult 'moment'. With her daughter, with her concerned colleagues, with parents on the gate and with both classes, her stress was affecting her body and now making it harder for people of all ages to feel safe with her – like a one-woman ripple affecting everyone she came into contact with.

Her realisation came tumbling out of her, among the group of other professionals she was with. She owned it. Her part. "It was all because of me," she acknowledged as she told her story. The group heard her. Her financial worries were the obvious root of it all. So were the ten years she had spent tiptoeing around her volcanic partner, the hidden side of her internal iceberg that she now realised was still tension – still energy – in her body and something she really wanted to be rid of.

She knew her financial concerns were not going away any time soon (short of a lottery win). What was in her control was her own body, and she determined then and there to become a more grounded, safer, version of herself. It might take a while, but she would benefit from this realisation, and those around her would, too.

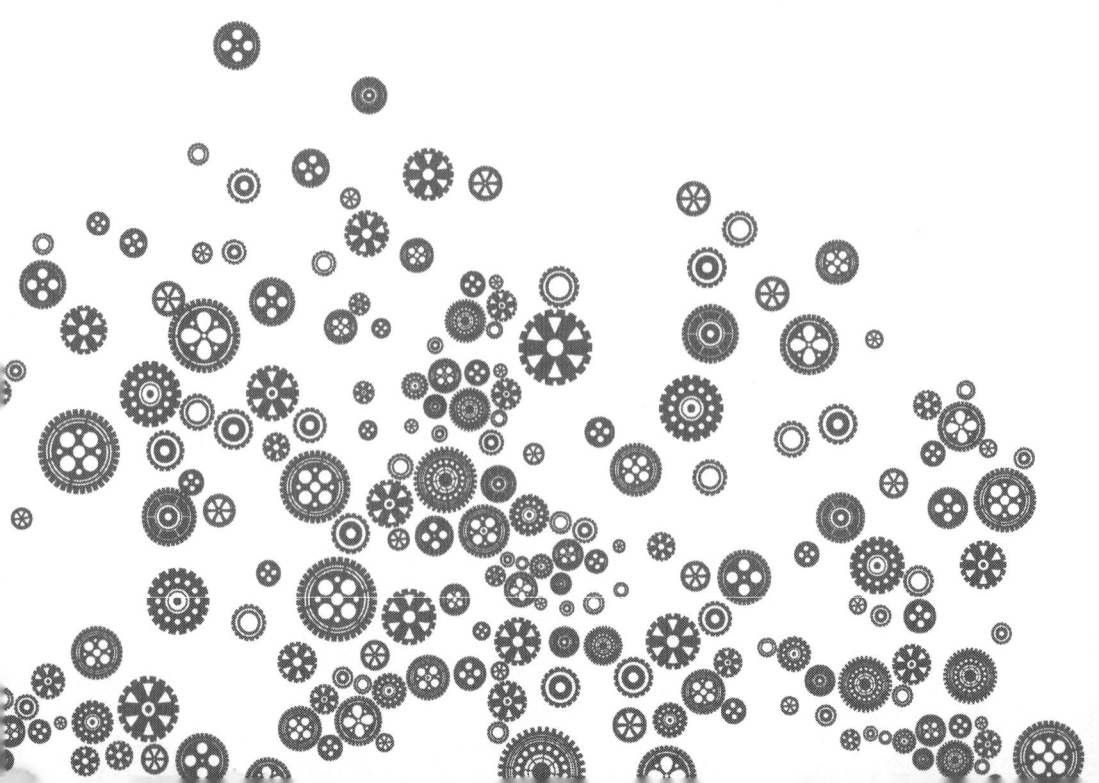

21

What Helps Us Get Grounded?

Having acknowledged that being grounded is more than just being calmer, calmer is a good place to start.

Things that can help us feel calmer … nicer … better can potentially start to shift our sympathetic nervous system (fight/flight) to our social engagement system and an increased sense of safety. There are many things that can do this, and the choice will be down to individual preference, but they can include the following.

Music

Singing – alone is good, with others even better!

Dancing (rhythmic movement)

Sitting on a swing (rhythmic movement)

Nature – walking (rhythmic movement), sitting and noticing

Breathing out (breathing in increases our heart rate, but breathing out slows it down – 'shhhhhh')

Being with safe people, making eye contact when you want to

Smiling – laughing; keep a few funny videos to hand, or a joke book

Stroking safe animals

Holding a calm/sleeping baby (human or animal)

Having a luxurious bath without being disturbed

Gardening

Laughing

Painting

Colouring

Rocking

Sitting on the floor

Lying on the floor on your back with your legs straight up the wall in front of you

Hanging upside-down in any way where your head is lower than your heart

Barefoot in the grass and sleeping babies may not be enough

Please know that none of these suggestions come with a guarantee.

It is very possible to do all these things, and become calmer or feel 'nicer', and yet still be in a dissociated state. It is perfectly possible for your nervous system to be in an 'activated' state when you go out for a walk in nature and still be in the same state when you come back.

The key is to really pay attention. Notice the slow breathing of a sleeping pet or baby and feel the weight of their body, notice where they are lying against you, and notice their smell.

Notice the feel of the soil – its temperature, texture, resistance to your spade – and the fragile petals or roots of whatever you are planting. Notice the parts of your body that you are using, and how they feel.

Notice the pattern of the thread on your car keys, following it with your finger and feeling the sensations of the ins and outs. Notice which parts of your body are involved in helping as you touch the key and notice how they all feel.

Right here, right now

The reality is that if we are around children – in our home or in a classroom – we often don't have time to just press 'pause' on life, take a nice leisurely stroll for ten minutes to smell the roses and feel our internal body sensations as we walk round the block alone, listening to the birds singing! The reality for us is that we are in the moment and we are responsible for what happens in this moment. We have to find a way to deal with things now, and what we really need to do is deal with ourselves now. Deal with our body. Deal with our nervous system.

Getting good at actually noticing when our nervous system is activated and when we are operating more from our 'mobilise' defensive set-up or our 'immobilise' shut-down set-up is a massive first step. If this has been our autopilot for years, possibly even decades, then it is a major deal to start to become conscious of ourselves. As you notice yourself in these states, please take at least half a moment to give yourself a silent (or out loud if you can) high-five! Becoming conscious and aware of what we have been doing unconsciously for years is growth, and always worth celebrating!

So then what? What else can we do that will help shift our nervous system down into a more grounded state? There are many other ways to help a body become grounded and start operating again from its social engagement system. The following are just a few. They include the ones I use myself and I have seen them all have almost immediate impact when I have shared them with clients of all ages. Generally, they only take a moment or two, and we can do all of these while still being 'in charge' of a classroom, siblings' mealtime, a football team or a carload of children.

1. Breathing out

Whatever breathing technique you use, the crucial element if you want to calm down is to make sure you breathe out for longer than you breathe in. Breathing in activates our sympathetic nervous system (fight/flight). It makes our heart beat faster, which is not helpful when we are trying to calm! Breathing out slows our heart rate and activates our restful parasympathetic nervous system.

One normal breath in and a very long one out can help change things quickly – especially if you repeat this a few times.

2. Use common senses

Using games that focus on the senses can help interrupt the activation of fight/flight set-up and can help us notice the (safe) environment we are in.

Find four things you can see that are blue

or

Find two things you can hear

or

Find something you like looking at

or

Take time to touch/stroke something that feels comforting, soothing, calming

The nerve endings in our fingertips are able to send a message to activate the release of serotonin. This is a feel-good hormone, which is why stroking a soft blanket, a furry animal or other calming textures can help us feel calmer.

3. Body sensations

The language of the deepest, oldest part of our brain is that of sensation in our body. Learning to notice our body sensations is, like noticing ourselves, a skill to be developed and mastered. However, in a moment when we need to bring ourselves into a grounded state, it is good to ask ourselves these questions, and really take as much time as we can to notice our body and find an answer before moving on.

Can you feel your shoulders? Are they up or down?

Notice the sensations as you put your feet in your shoes. What do they feel like?

Notice the sensations as you hold your hand under a tap of running water. Does it feel nice to you?

Notice the sensations as you hold a book, a ball, an apple or a pencil. How would you describe them?

Notice and follow the sensation as the water in the shower hits your head or shoulder and runs down from there. Can you trace the water? Do you resist it or welcome the feeling of it?

4. Connection

Noticing our internal body sensations right here and now, and combining them with where we connect to something that is solid and supporting us, can help to bring in the crucial element and depth of *grounded-ness*.

Can you feel your feet on the floor? What does the floor feel like? Do your feet like that feeling? Now notice how solid the floor is to support you and hold you up.

or

Notice how soft the carpet is, to give you comfort, and yet how strong the floor is, to hold you up.

or

Notice how your back feels being supported by that chair ...

Notice all the parts of your body that are in contact with that chair/table/etc., supporting you/holding you up. What does it feel like?

5. Smile

The muscles in our face are closely connected with the muscles in our middle ear. When we do not feel safe, and our middle ear moves to help us detect and locate the low frequencies around us, the muscles around our eyes and in our cheeks also change very quickly into a facial expression of worry or anger or just impassivity.

If we can make ourselves smile, we can almost reverse-engineer the situation, and show our brain that we are smiling and therefore not really under threat.

6. Sit or lie down on the floor

Sometimes when our nervous system gets activated into a fight/flight or shut-down state, we can feel quite exposed standing up. Simply moving to sit on the floor, perhaps leaning against a wall or strong chair, and feeling the solidity of the floor supporting us can be a really powerful way to change the energy and therefore the brain message in our body.

Getting down on the floor in the middle of a 'moment' with a child at home can be extra beneficial by surprising the child (they weren't expecting you to do this) and decreasing any threat element they are feeling from your body being bigger than theirs. In the classroom, for teachers who are up and on their feet most of the day, actually sitting down on the carpet with their class or even just a few pupils and taking a few seconds to really notice their connection with the floor can be a lovely, subtle way to help their own body feel supported and safer again without interrupting the flow of a lesson.

There have been many occasions in my career when I have been in a room with children bursting with huge emotional energy – and even more times when I have been with irate adults. Sometimes it has been parents who are desperate because they don't understand their child or there is a breakdown of trust with the school. Sometimes it has been school staff, lunchtime supervisors, teaching assistants, teachers and headteachers, who are fuming for any one of a number of reasons. My go-to, in-the-moment combination for keeping myself grounded, even though my nervous system is trying to respond to their anger and push me into defensive mode, is a powerful one–two combo.

1. I feel myself strongly connecting with my chair. I put some brain attention into noticing my bottom on the chair, pushing my back into its back and feeling strongly supported by it.

2. I smile. Finding a way to do this without the irate person thinking I am smiling *at them* is always achievable. I start smiling and the muscles in my face, my eyes and mouth change. The configuration sends a message to the safety-detection part of my brain that 'she is smiling – she must be OK; it's OK – we don't need to leave, we can stay here and we don't have to get aggressive, either'.

The person I am with has no idea what is going on inside me, as I work internally with myself, my body and my face. They just get to see my safe smile, and will detect me as a calm, grounded, safe, supportive person who is with them in a non-threatening way.

Getting grounded is a sound investment

When you can fully feel your internal body sensations (your interoception, as Porges would call it), as well as use other senses to notice what is happening around you in your environment and with other people if they are present, then you are most likely 'grounded'. If we need to take a couple of moments to

1. move into another room

2. face a different direction, or simply

3. stop and become aware of ourselves and our bodies,

while we focus internally for a few moments, these will always be moments well spent. Whatever time we use getting ourselves grounded will never be time wasted. In fact, it will be time that we invest in seeing - and creating - better outcomes. When we are grounded we will be able to help situations improve rather than stay the same or get worse.

22

Getting Grounded, Wrapping Presents

Working in a school suited Rachel. She loved kids, loved seeing them grow and become more of their best selves. Of course, there were the usual things that didn't thrill her, but for the most part there was something every day that filled her deepest place.

Conscientious and hard-working, she always arrived in the mornings with plenty of time before any meetings she might have, and certainly before there was any sound of children – which worked in her favour this particular morning.

Her 'get up – get ready' routine had gone as normal and, just before she left home, there was an argument with her partner. Nothing that unusual there. The arguments had been a regular feature recently. Feeling her body tighten as it braced itself against every word he shouted at and about her, she could only think about one thing: get out of the house. This was progress in itself. In the past she had lived so much in the freeze state that the shouting used to completely disable her. She would collapse on the inside and find it really hard to think, or even move. Something like this could have had her unplugged for the whole day – or longer.

But she was growing and changing, and today's response was different: keep moving and get away from the onslaught. In her car she would be alone, she would be safe. Her vision went funny as she came down the stairs to the door; she could still see, but it was odd – smaller, somehow, and blurry around the edges. She realised that arrows were still being shouted at her, but she couldn't hear them. Her hearing had changed too, and it didn't bother her one bit – she was on mission 'get away'. Slamming the front door felt so good – in the past she'd been too afraid to make a noise when she felt vulnerable. Not today. She loved the slam; it helped say something she couldn't, yet, but it didn't calm her down. She fumbled with her keys. Her hands were shaking and didn't seem to have their usual dexterity.

The first set of traffic lights were on red. It was a long line of cars; she would be there a while. She joined the queue and put her car into neutral, accepting the enforced break in her fleeing. She realised she had done it – she had got away, and she was safe. She noticed herself. The tightness in her muscles reduced a little bit, enough that she could take her first proper breath in and out since it all began. And then came the wave she wasn't expecting. Emotions washed over and through her like an unexpected tide. When she was in freeze or dissociated, she didn't feel things – which at times like this, she thought, had its benefits. Now she was able to mobilise herself to get away from threat and get herself to safety, and it meant her emotions were mobilised, too – she was starting to feel things. As the tears started to gush down her face, she knew she had a choice: carry on to school and try her old technique of stuffing herself, her feelings and her response back inside like a sleeping bag being stuffed back into a tight cover; or do something different.

She knew she wasn't grounded. She knew what would probably happen for the rest of the day if she took her ungrounded nervous system into the school building. She knew how the sensitive children she worked with would pick up on her dysregulation, be unsettled by it, struggle, and then get told off for their behaviour. Even other staff she worked with, some of whom were less-than-grounded themselves, would likely unconsciously react to her; however much she could try to placate them with her familiar 'I'm OK', 'business as usual' attitude, their nervous systems would pick up on hers and they might get even more short with the children. It wouldn't go well. She also knew it would be harder for her to get herself grounded again in that environment. She was still learning these skills and, being so activated this morning, her nervous system needed some respect. She made a choice, took responsibility for herself and turned her car round. She had time. She went back home, where she was now alone in the house.

Even just stepping through the door, she felt a bit better – proud of herself, even. It was new to be noticing herself and choosing to do what she needed to do to be safe. It was new choosing to put herself and her nervous system first, instead of pushing through, denying, pretending, dissociating. She sat on the bottom stair and howled. The tears and anger gushed from her. She allowed herself to give full expression to this pain. She knew it was not only from the shouting that morning, but some of the pain she had stuffed, suppressed and dissociated from for decades. For just that moment, she allowed herself to honour it, to feel it, to let it be.

In a few moments it was done. There were no more tears. She quietened. Her head seemed clearer. She could still feel the adrenaline in her body, her heart was galloping, and her legs felt more like those of a newborn foal when she stood up. She was better, but still not grounded. She was still not ready to go and face the day in school and she still had time on her side. She made a quick scan of her mental to-do list, to use the extra time she had at home well. The list was long, but she knew all the jobs that required proper brain power were no-go. She needed something easy.

The end of term was coming, it would soon be Christmas and she had gifts to wrap for other staff. She set about this job she enjoyed doing at the best of times. Moving her hands slowly and simply, manipulating nothing more than paper, scissors, sticky tape and ribbon, she made things that looked beautiful. Matching the colours of paper and ribbon seemed to soothe her. Listening to the sound of the ribbon pulling against the scissor blade before it sprang into ringlets was reassuring. Her hearing and sight were fully back to normal. Thinking about the person each gift was for, what she was grateful for about them and the enjoyment she would have giving these gifts out, brought a smile back to her face and to her soul. Now she was ready.

23

What's In A Smile?

Smiling got a mention in Chapter 21 as one of my personal go-to strategies for helping my body to get grounded when I am in a potentially threatening environment – especially when it is a professional situation and, although I might feel extremely uncomfortable internally, I know with my cognitive, rational brain, that I am actually safe.

Smiling is powerful, and something we need to look at a bit more.

Smiling affects all the muscles in our face and, crucially, our inner ear. It is something we can only do authentically when we feel grounded and safe. It is interesting, though, that if we put our face muscles into a smile, even when we don't feel like it, 90% of the time it doesn't take our brains very long to process the smiling face, interpret this as a signal of being safe and help relax the rest of our body – and, all of a sudden, we are actually smiling for real.

> **Try this:** You can try this out by holding a pencil or pen sideways in your mouth, so that it pushes your cheeks into the shape of a smile. Make sure it is as far back in your teeth as possible and see how long it is before those cheeks are smiling even if you take the pen away.

When we are with another person, especially a child, who is themselves dysregulated in their body, we need to understand that our face is the purveyor of multiple meanings.

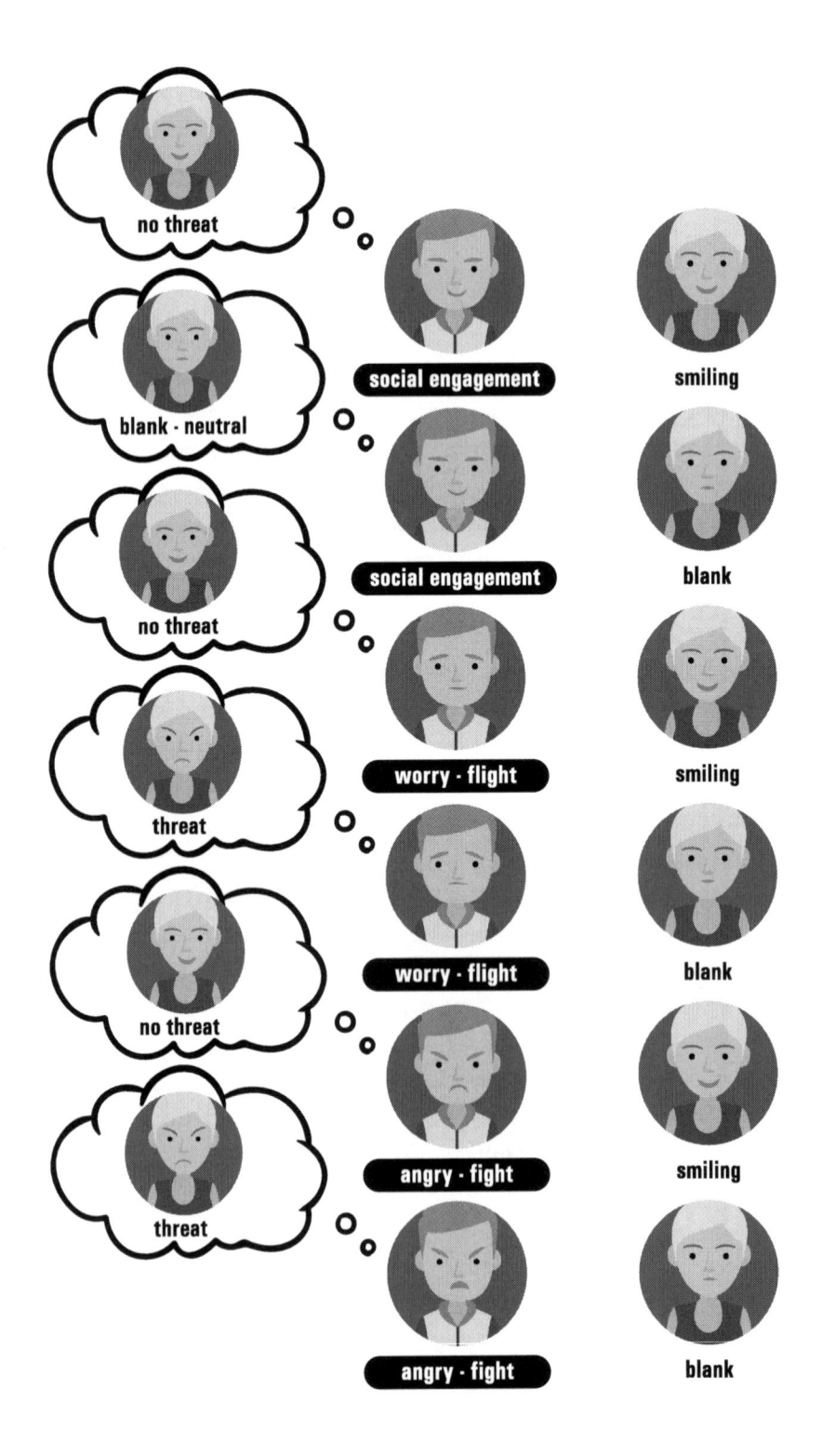

Thought	Perceived face	Actual face
no threat	social engagement	smiling
blank - neutral	social engagement	blank
no threat	worry - flight	smiling
threat	worry - flight	blank
no threat	angry - fight	smiling
threat	angry - fight	blank

Worrying about blank faces

Emma was an anxious girl. One of the top set groups, she was always trying her best. She worked hard at her work, and with those around her; she was desperate to keep the peace as much as she could, whether she was with friends on the playground, at gymnastics or minding her little brother and his mates. At school she liked her teacher and was glad to be in her class. However, she would frequently ask her teacher if she was OK. "Are you OK, Mrs Harris?" became one of the familiar phrases that the teacher would need to respond to several times a week. By coincidence, it became apparent that Emma regularly asked this of certain other members of staff, too. What could be driving this repeated question? Was she looking for attention? Was she hoping for an opening where she could be of help? Did she want to get closer to her teacher in some way?

The confusion only intensified when her teacher asked her about her questioning. "Emma, I'm curious to know what it is about me that makes you need to ask me if I am OK." Emma, wanting to get the answer right, blurted the clearest answer she could muster: "Umm, you don't seem OK". When she was reassured by Mrs Harris that she – and, in fact, everything right then – was OK, Emma was able to find more words. She explained, "Most of the time you have a pretty face – you smile a lot when you are talking to us. It makes you look pretty. Sometimes you don't seem OK, though – you don't have your pretty smile and you make me think you are cross."

Emma's teacher had a beautiful demeanour. She was calm and quiet, yet firm when she needed to be, and was sensitive to and really cared about her class. She realised what Emma was saying was that when she was smiling, everything was OK for Emma. However, when, for those moments in a day, she happened to have a straight face, Emma really struggled and thought she was angry. Was she really supposed to be walking around smiling 24/7 when she was at school? How could a child who was so bright and clever at school – so anxious to get things right – get it so wrong, thinking she was angry when she was just thinking, or waiting, or ...?

As we can see from the diagram, a child already subconsciously feeling unsafe within their nervous system and internal physiology – which is true for all quietly anxious children as well as the obviously upset ones – will struggle to read a blank face as just a blank face. Instead they will interpret it as threatening more danger. Not surprisingly, then, there is even more reason for us to understand why children sometimes choose to keep their distance from us when they are struggling and we just want to help.

This is something I have had to work on to develop for myself. I was always referred to as a 'serious, sensible little girl' at school. What my infant and junior teachers were seeing all those years ago was that my face went 'blank' and even into a bit of a frown when I was really concentrating. Being aware that this can still happen (even though I am in schools for a whole different reason now) has really helped me. I notice when I feel myself concentrating and realise my face is not being at all helpful to the person/people I am with, who is/are struggling emotionally at that moment. I know how to change that instantly – and I find a way to smile. I want to make sure that, as far as I am able, they do not perceive my face – i.e. me – as a threat to them at a time when they don't feel safe in the world.

24

Changing The Landscape

With so many diverse ways to help ourselves get grounded and bring our nervous system into an 'I am safe' state of play, it may appear easy.

Sometimes it is instinctive: 'I'm going for a walk/run', or grabbing a crunchy apple and eating it outside on a swing (while paying attention to the crunch, taste and swallow, the birds singing and the sensations in your body swinging back and forth). But it may not be. In the heat of an activated nervous system, it takes significantly increased self-awareness to consciously notice what is going on inside. Our tendency is to get carried away with thoughts and emotion, to 'go into our heads', often disconnecting from what is happening in our body. Being aware of what is going on in our body is even harder if we are living in a highly activated state, where fight, flight or shut-down patterns have become our 'normal'. It is important that *each one of us takes time to find out which techniques work for us and builds our own personal tool kit.* We can become responsible for ourselves and equipped to help ourselves get grounded, wherever and whenever we need to.

If we begin to realise that, more often than not, we are living in a high-stress state, have pain in our body (particularly back, shoulder, neck or joint pain), have sleep issues, digestive issues or a short fuse, and/or are frequently irritable or anxious, we may need to help ourselves – help our bodies – in a more significant way than by just using the occasional grounding 'tools'.

The list of traumatic experiences in Chapter 20 is not exhaustive. There could be other ways in which a nervous system was squeezed so hard by life that it became overwhelmed. If this has been the case, it is no surprise to find a nervous system still operating in a state of high activation where the sympathetic nervous system is still driving fight/

flight survival patterns, or the dorsal vagus nerve of the parasympathetic nervous system is still helping us immobilise and hide from life, years after the horrible experience(s).

What we need to understand in these situations is that it is more likely that the nervous system has got 'stuck' in the different survival states. Instead of processing the huge energy surge from the survival moment and then coming back to a grounded, calm, safe state after the event, our body kept going and going and going, and then, before long, that level of activation became the new 'normal'. Having adrenaline pumping, a faster heart rate, tight muscles and shallower breathing became so usual and familiar that they don't seem strange any more. In fact, for many people who live this way – and believe me, there are many – actually feeling still, calm, safe and totally relaxed in their body is really, really strange at first.

It is worth mentioning at this point that your body's ability to relax fully, to feel totally safe and to be grounded has nothing to do with your age, your abilities, your profession, your level of spirituality or your health. Having worked with little people, mature people, brilliant minds, people at the top of their professional 'pole' and those with fitness levels many of us would envy, I can assure you that the fact remains: when the body – the nervous system – is overwhelmed by one-off or long-term stressors it will be affected, and the impact can last … for a lifetime, if not helped to recover fully.

Stress in the body
Stress from trauma or long-term overwhelming situations can eventually start to show up within the body as symptoms of one of many physical conditions. While certain GPs still do not understand the links, thankfully there are increasing numbers of functional medical practitioners who do. These are professionals in the medical field who aim to treat their patients with an integrative approach and to help them regain health, instead of just manage disease. These practitioners appreciate that the impact of stress and trauma on a body can be significant. They understand that often just talking to a friend, counsellor or even a therapist does not bring enough change to the nervous system, which is at

the root of where the change needs to happen. Healing the body often starts with restoring safety in the nervous system.

> Marilyn is a grandma. She dotes on her grandchildren and loves having time with them whenever they visit. She barely left her house, and only came to see me when she was desperate to finally emerge from a two-year life-shrinking sentence of severe anxiety and depression. She was on all sorts of medication and the biggest thing that bothered her was the way her body shook. She would shake when she was sitting watching TV, when she was on the phone, and even when she was trying to go to sleep. She just couldn't seem to make it stop, and even the drugs her doctor prescribed didn't seem to have the same effect any more.
>
> The story of Marilyn's life, which came out in snippets over the course of her sessions, was one of multiple hardships, heartache and trauma among the joys. Now in her 70s, she spoke indirectly and very briefly of two occasions when bad things happened to her as a little girl. Talking about what she'd experienced wasn't part of what was needed, but it was something she wanted me to know, because she had never told anyone else. She had just kept those horrible feelings inside her and not mentioned anything to anyone – for decades. She understood completely how her body had stored the tension from those experiences and how life, over the many years since, had compiled the tension in her internal muscles. She understood that her nervous system had responded back then to try and help her survive, but that she now needed some help to get back to 'normal operations' again.
>
> A few sessions of learning a new way to work with her body was what it took for her to start to reclaim her life. Her body was becoming more still. She was feeling 'her old self' and smiling again. She came triumphantly to her fourth session announcing to me that 'this thing you're teaching me, dear, it's working!'

TRE

The 'thing' Marilyn was learning was a tool that many people of all ages have found to be helpful for down-regulating an overactive nervous system: a technique called TRE (Tension Releasing Exercises). This is a non-verbal way of releasing tension held in the body and changing the internal landscape of the body and the nervous system from one of stress, tension and high activation to one of calm, safety and more appropriate responses in the nervous system.

TRE is a beautiful way to down-regulate your autonomic nervous system, by focusing initially on the psoas muscles, which many people now understand to be a significant muscle group that tightens when we are stressed or overwhelmed or experience trauma of any sort. Some people call it our 'stress or survival muscle'. The psoas major runs from the tops of our thighs through our hips and pelvic bone and connects to the first five vertebrae at the bottom of our spine. It holds tension for a long time – days, weeks, months, years and even decades. Long-held tension in the psoas is often the cause of lower back pain. Tension in this area is also known to be linked to a poor parasympathetic response – so the more we can help this muscle release its tension, the more we strengthen our ability to rest, relax and restore. The tension of surviving is held encased in this muscle, so it is no surprise that when it starts to relax again we can find our social engagement 'safety' set-up more quickly, along with improved digestion and relaxed facial muscles.

TRE works by helping the body naturally activate neurogenic tremors. Essentially it is a safe way to help the human body to do what animals do instinctively. When there is stress or threat of any sort, an animal will 'shake it off' when it is safe again. Watch the next time your dog has to do something it doesn't enjoy: a car ride, meeting dominating or unfriendly dogs, nail-clipping, a trip to the vets or learning to wear a car harness can all be followed by a quick shake. When horses have fallen, the first thing they do when they get up is send a shudder down through the muscles in their body. Google 'polar bear trauma' and you'll see a video of how shaking to de-stress is an instinctive response of polar bears, too. We can do the same – once we get over our Western mindset that says tremoring or shaking in any way is wrong or bad or a sign of weakness, that is. Many people have found that, after decades of suffering and taking themselves through years of talking and other therapies, TRE has been the way to actually change their body from the inside out, in ways they couldn't possibly have imagined.

TRE is best learnt with the support of a trained and experienced TRE provider. Going at the right pace for you is crucial. Feeling totally safe throughout the experience leads to fruitful healing experiences. Many people benefit from help in finding their best speed by working with a grounded, experienced practitioner. Some providers are also experienced therapists and have a deeper understanding of trauma and keeping clients safe. If that is important to you, then you can choose. You may only need a few one-to-one sessions to learn the process safely for your body, or you may benefit from working with a professional for longer. If you want to find out more about TRE, and find a list of qualified practitioners, check out the websites listed in the Additional Resources section.

Grounding

No book called *Grounded* and looking at how we can become calmer human beings can go without mentioning the term 'grounding' in its other context! There is an emerging body of evidence that connecting with the earth can have a discharging effect on our bodies. It works on the understanding that our bodies carry an electrical charge, which is released or neutralised when we walk barefoot on the earth – the ground outside. The principle is the same as the way that a lightning rod on the side of a building can help direct the electrical charge from the sky safely into the ground.

The length of time many of us spend outside with shoes off in the summer, and how much better we feel for it, is being used as one example of how effective this mode of 'discharging' ourselves is. Spending time walking barefoot in the grass was recommended to me during a health retreat that I went on several year ago in Mexico. It was easy to feel calmer and less 'charged' doing this on the gorgeous thick grass there, on the edge of the coast with the sound of the sea in the background and the pelicans flying overhead. For me the benefits became more apparent when I returned to the UK. Reconnecting with my 'normal' life was a much better way to notice the calming benefits I felt from continuing this practice.

Sadly, living where I do, the reality is that getting my shoes off and spending time wandering around my garden barefoot (among the slugs and in the cold, rain and snow!) is a stressful thought in itself for a large part of the year! For those who have the budget for shoes and mattresses that help to conduct our increased electrical charge away from our body and into the ground, these may be additional methods to consider.

Somatic Experiencing

Similarly to TRE, Somatic Experiencing, or Somatic Practice, is based on the understanding that animals in the wild frequently experience life-threatening moments and yet don't seem to get traumatised by them. They have an instinctive way to release the extra energy from their body naturally after the threat has passed. Humans, however, often do not finish the cycle the way animals do, so the energy never gets dissipated and is trapped in our bodies. Somatic therapies focus on how the trauma has been trapped in the body. It will focus on both cognitive (mind) and body work. It will help a person to restore the balance to their autonomic nervous system as well as remember and psychologically resolve the traumatic situation so it loses its intensity. This does not involve 'reliving' the trauma but, rather, reviewing the events around it (before and after). As with TRE, if this is a practice that you are interested in exploring, the best advice is to always work with an experienced, qualified practitioner.

Advice to anyone thinking about starting therapy ... of any sort

1. If you ever find yourself meeting someone for the first time who has the credentials to see you through a journey of healing (mind, body or spirit), please, please, please *trust your instincts*. If you do not feel safe *in every way* with them when you meet, your journey with them will be a superficial one at best, a waste of time on average, and more damaging to you at worst.

2. Please vote with your feet and, if you are not comfortable and don't feel you can challenge the practitioner, just *don't go back*. You don't need to. It's about getting *you* the right help match for *you*. You could either *ask for a different professional from the same organisation* to work with or *go somewhere completely different*.

3. *See your first meeting as an interview or audition* – and it's not you that's on trial, but the professional. If they don't meet the simple and appropriate criteria of making you feel *safe, heard, respected and understood*, or if anything feels 'off' to you, then just be grateful you didn't go any further down the line with them and move on.

I fully understand that it takes some real emotional energy to do this – it can be much easier to go along with what the 'professional' says. However, I think many people don't realise that you can and *should* have a voice and need to *opt in* to working with someone you feel will be a good match for you. As we have learnt from Dr Porges, we can use our neuroception – we know when we feel safe with someone. And we know when we don't.

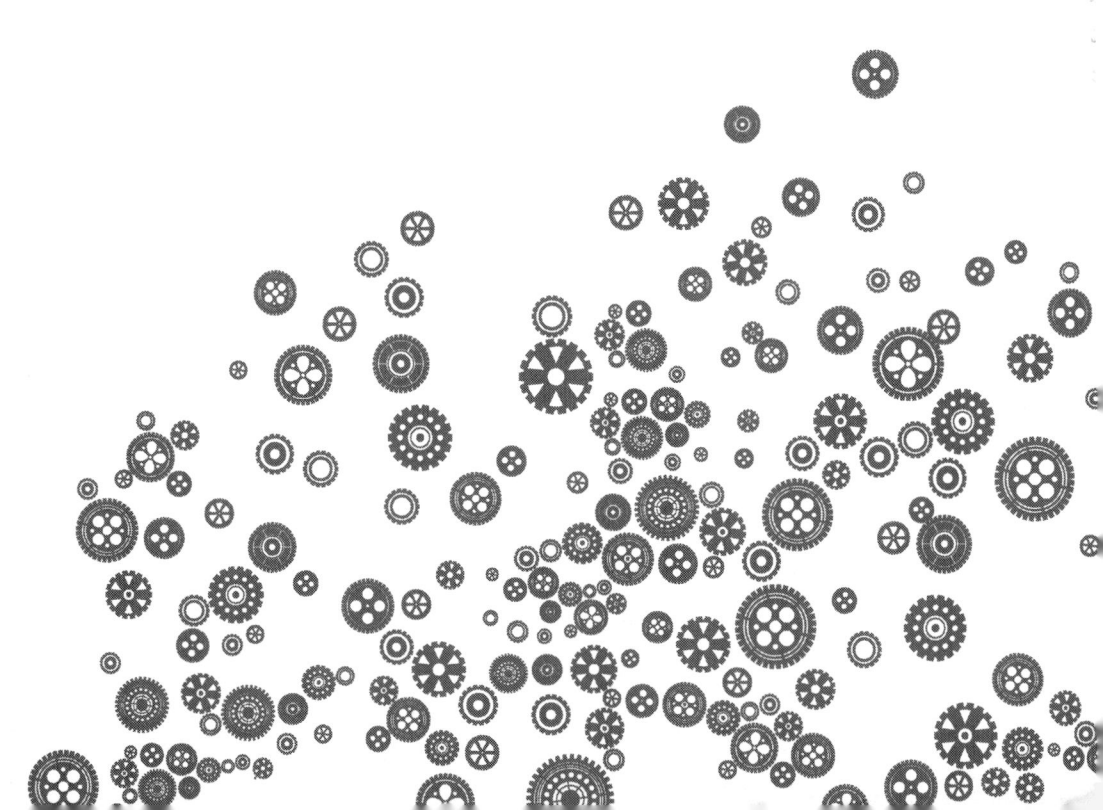

SECTION 4

HOPE

Children are the living messages we send to a time we will not see.

Neil Postman

Do the best you can until you know better. Then when you know better, do better.

Maya Angelou

When little people are overwhelmed by big emotions it is our job to share our calm, not join their chaos.

L.R. Knost

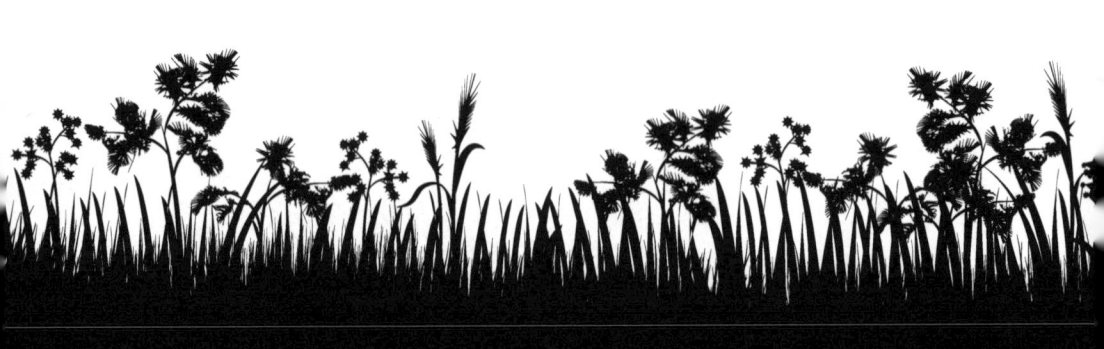

25

The Benefits Of Grounded Adults

Children know if they are safe with us. They know from our faces, our body tension, our movement, our gestures, our eyes and eyebrows, our mouths and our speech. If we are not safe for them, as their neuroception registers it in a particular moment, they will need to protect themselves and their neurophysiology will change, as we have already explored – and all this without them 'consciously' realising.

Detecting safety

As a reminder, these are the main ways their eyes and ears will be detecting whether we are grounded, and therefore safe. They will be watching and listening to subconscious messages from our:

Body language

Hand gestures

Tone

Volume

Intonation

Speed

Facial expression

Muscle tension

Eye contact

However, if a child is experiencing threat from something in their environment, it is important to realise they will be taking increasing cues from us. If they are scared of a spider, for example, and we are also scared of the spider, we are no help! Our nervous system activation, muscle tension, flappy hands, screechy voice, rushing and odd behaviour will let them know that yes, we are scared too, and so they are totally spot-on to be frightened!

If they are scared and we are really scared but we pretend not to be, it is likely we will still be little help in calming them. Why? Because *bodies speak louder than words*. The child will be able to detect an incongruence in our body and voice. The message our body is giving ('*not* safe') will be at odds with the message we are telling them in words ("There's nothing to worry about").

However, if they are scared and we are totally safe and grounded and have an integrity to our body and voice, we will be able to help them come out of their 'danger' state. It may even be that, due to our 'this is no threat to me' cues, the child may, given time, be able to calm enough to help us catch the spider and look at it up-close. They may be able to marvel at it through the upturned glass before they help us, calmly, release it safely outside.

Let's remember that, just like James doing his homework (Chapter 17), if the child feels unsafe with us in this moment, the spider will be a second threat and the child will be having to survive their fear on their own. In the same way, if a child has worries about something, or has experienced something that is bothering them, but they detect we are not safe right in that moment, they will not come near us to talk about it. In this circumstance, however much we tell a child they can and should come to us if anything is bothering them, we need to recognise their neuroception and realise that how safe they feel we are will be the deciding factor on whether they obey us or not.

We can only be a help to them if we are not also a subconscious threat. It is only when we are grounded that we can fully help a child to calm.

The technical term for when our very presence and interaction can help calm another whose nervous system is more aroused (scared/angry/anxious or hyper/excited) is *co-regulation*. As we realised from Dr

Perry, co-regulation is the first stage in helping to bring the best out of children. Our *biggest tool is our own body*. Through our nervous system, our body keeps communicating that we are safe and therefore things are OK: 'I am safe and I can help you feel calm again'. A cuddle, a hug, sitting side-by-side or on the floor back-to-back, doing something as simple as swaying with rhythm or movement, in silence or with gentle conversation with another, can help the dysregulated child's heart rate come into sync with the calmer adult's heartbeat. Breathing slows, muscles relax and in a short time safety physiology is resumed. Sometimes, who we are – our very essence – is the biggest gift we can offer to help another.

Sometimes just being close and speaking gently with another is all we need to do for them to see the safety in our face, hear the calmness in our tone of voice, and for their subconscious to process all the information they get from our calm, relaxed body so that they too can calm again. They have choices and, if they don't detect that safety from us, they will probably act to confront us or get away.

What if I really am scared of spiders? Then what do I do?

If you are genuinely scared of spiders, the best way to help a child is to be honest with them, while still doing everything you can to help yourself stay as grounded as possible, using the tools in Chapter 21. Imagine saying to a child:

> Oh my word, yup, it's a spider and you know I don't like spiders very much ... but listen, I am going to get control of my body so I can stay calm, and then I will be able to use my brain properly and figure out the best way to help us all (spider included!) to be OK.

This approach will bring the authenticity the child needs to hear – and they will probably trust you to do what you said. They will understand any tension or fear they detect from you because they know you are actually a bit scared. What you are saying to them lets them know that you are in charge, you have a plan ... and they will watch (and learn) as you role-model your way into dealing with one of your fears. What an incredible lesson to give them! The more children can observe their adults manage themselves when they get dysregulated, the quicker they will learn how to do it too.

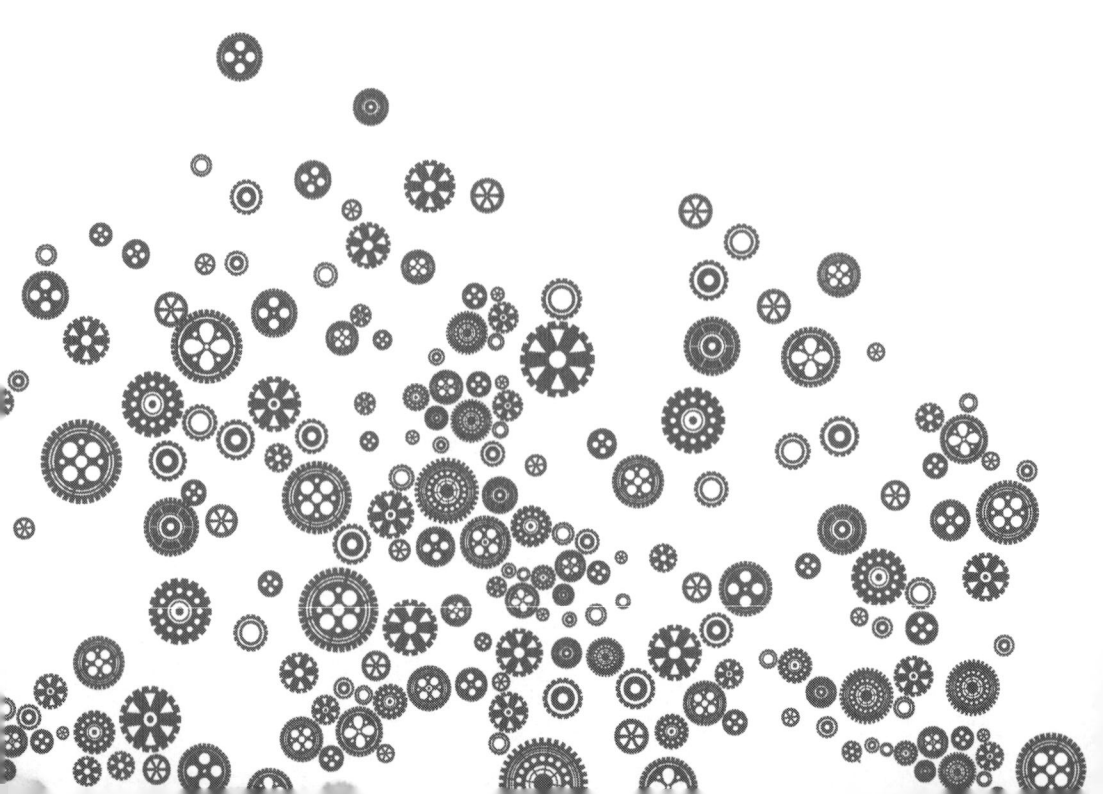

26

Supporting Narnia's Children

Grounded grown-ups are very powerful to scared, angry, threatened or overwhelmed children. The very presence of a grounded, caring adult can start to heal the most damaged child. It may be slow work, but it will be worth it when you start to see the glimpses of personality coming out, just like the first hints of the black, beady eyes and shiny black nose of the little hedgehog face as she slowly detects that, here and now, with this person, "I am safe to come out of my shut-down spiky ball".

> Oliver was hanging on by a thread. He was using all his survival skills as best his six-year-old subconscious brain and body knew how. He had been living in high-level un-safety ever since he was born.
>
> For Oliver, home was chaotic: shouting, inconsistency, danger, high emotions, vibes, threat. Chaos was his 'normal'. *Not* feeling safe was his 'everyday', his 'typical'. To his nervous system, 'home = unsafe = hard work'. He needed to be on alert the whole time. He had had several experiences that really scared him when he was tiny, including getting trapped in a box – from which he managed to escape by getting his toddler body climbing up, up, up and breaking through the top.
>
> In his few short years, he had never experienced what it felt like to feel safe. Not really. Not on the inside of himself ... and now was no exception. He was older, but things still happened at home that really scared him. He stayed frozen, functioning just as much as he needed to in order to hang on – making smaller and smaller movements, not making any eye contact, hardly speaking. Life was exclusively about survival. His instincts kept him alive and he unknowingly excelled in hiding, not being noticed, and not feeling anything. Like one of the frozen statues in Narnia, he felt nothing and this was the best way.

At school, things were hard. The lights, the bodies, the noise ... it was too much for his brain to process and it all confirmed to him his need to stay in shut-down/freeze. Work was hard, too. It also felt like a threat. His emotional brain was functioning around the age of three, while his body was in a class of six-year-olds. When he had to do work, he struggled so much he would feel like (and his body would respond like) he was in danger all over again.

Safety in a grown-up body
The good news for Oliver was his support lady. She stuck by him and, although sometimes she didn't really fully get him, he knew she liked him. He didn't know *how* he knew – because having someone enjoy him was a new and weird experience for him – but somehow he did. He enjoyed her smile. He enjoyed her being around for him. He enjoyed the sparkle in her eyes and the gentle way she spoke to him. He started to feel a bit different. Where people at home felt like tsunamis, she felt like a millpond. Where they were raging storms, she was like gentle, soft spring rain that falls silently and soaks into your clothes and gets to your skin without you even thinking you are getting wet.

Oliver's nervous system started to detect there was less threat to his life when she was around. It started slowly to thaw from its complex freeze. When they come out of freeze, all bodies head back into the big energies of the mobilising stages they were in before the final overwhelm and shut-down happened. Oliver was just the same. Lashing out and running became frequent expressions of his body. His muscles had held in their tension from not being able to fight or get away to safety for so many years. Those around him who only saw the behaviour thought it was bad news. They didn't understand that his climbing up fences was in fact his body still trying to finish surviving what had happened in that box when he was three, and all the other times he really wanted to get away to get safe. Why would they? Many of them didn't even know that part of his story – and, anyway, it was a long time ago now, surely he would have forgotten ...

Healing trauma can be a messy journey

Oliver's healing process, itself an indicator that he was feeling safer, was actually now making him harder to 'manage'. His new internal experiences of strong emotions made his body need to move, to 'mobilise', to flight. His running came from his new-found sense of being safe. He felt safer now, with his special safe lady near him. His conscious mind would not necessarily recall the experience from three years before, but his body, just like all bodies, remembered. His body was trying to complete discharging the energy and physical movements that he hadn't been able to complete back then, and all of this while trying to navigate numeracy, phonics and silent reading. He felt safer than he ever had been, and it was getting him into so much trouble.

The mindset that says 'when children start to heal, they should become "easier"' and 'when children feel safe they should behave in a calm way' was leading staff to think they were not helping him at all. In fact, the opposite was true. The next bit of learning for all the staff at school was the lesson Oliver was showing them. Children (and adults) who have experienced complex trauma and been in freeze for years can start to heal – but only as they feel safe to do so – if the adults around them are grounded enough. Navigating safely the energies of suppressed anger (fight) and fear (flight) will be the next stage in the healing journey, and a time when those surrounding adults need to work hard to hold on to their own grounded-ness, for their sake and the child's.

27

What Children Want

We live at a time when many people are starting to realise how important it is that we *take children seriously*. The statistics about children's mental health are alarming, and my sense is that the numbers still only scratch the surface of the magnitude of suffering our young people are enduring.

In schools more and more 'behaviour policies' are being revamped in an attempt to find some way of keeping up with the wide and varied behaviours children are displaying in the classroom – and 'policy-fy' them. Many caring and conscientious schools are desperate to find a way to do this that takes account of the wide-ranging situations the children live in, acknowledges the range of mental health conditions they have already been diagnosed with, and honours the multiple reasons behind different behaviours.

Despite the current financial climate, many parents are still doing their best to give their child 'the best'. The best clothes, shoes and technology. The best trips, toys and holidays. Children want the best. For sure, they love it when they get special things but, when it comes down to it, when the rubber really hits the road, they want the best 'us'.

> I was working with 60 eight-year-olds recently and our final session together was a time I will not forget. As well as sharing their celebration stories and their highlights of our time together, they stung me with their honest desperation. It came as a quiet plea: please will you do these sessions for our parents, too? One girl spoke of her mum, how she worried a lot and sometimes cried, and she wanted her to feel calmer. A boy told me how his dad was angry – he didn't know what about, but he wanted him to be able to get more grounded. *Children notice who*

we are, and they worry about us. What they want the most is for the key adults in their world – their most important people – to be calm, to be grounded, and to be OK again.

If we were to risk really paying attention to the children, we might realise that, in this time of desperately grasping for mental health solutions for so many children, we have an answer. We, in fact, *are* an answer. Please understand that I am not suggesting it is all down to us. I am not suggesting that, by becoming generations of grounded parents, teachers, grandparents, Scout leaders, football coaches, music teachers and gym instructors we will eradicate all the mental health issues our children contend with. No. I *am* saying, though, that what the children themselves seem to be asking for matches up with what Stephen Porges meant when he said that our "most profound and intervening variable is our own physiological state".

Doing something about that is a journey only each of us can choose to take. It is our own choice for who we want to be. We may not have the capacity to change the whole world for all children. But we can begin the journey to change ourselves and our world – and change the experience of the children around us.

28

Jane's Special Story

Jane is the mother of a child with a rare genetic condition. Life caring for and advocating for her daughter through those years of childhood and adolescence was incredibly hard in every possible way. Not surprisingly, she used to get stressed out and exhausted very easily. This is what she told me.

> Yes, I had feelings – so many feelings! They ranged from disappointment to real anger, and they were often lurking at the edges of every day, ready to pounce! It was interesting, though, you know, that once I took some of the focus off my child and started to focus some of my attention on myself, things started to change. Once I learnt to be more calm and to assist my internal reactions to settle, when I wanted to just blow, I actually got less and less reactive. It sounds weird to say it, but I guess I got less angry in my body.
>
> Other people I know who had similarly challenging experiences of parenting a child with complex special needs seemed calm, but in a different way. They seemed like they just weren't quite there anymore. They were so physically and emotionally spent, and so used to those massive feelings not getting them anywhere, they just got quiet inside – like apathetic – overwhelmed.
>
> As for me, though, I worked hard at helping myself with the little bits of energy I had. I learnt TRE and used all sorts of other techniques, and really discovered what I was like, who I was, when I was less reactive and more grounded. And that's when it got even more interesting!
>
> With me being calmer around my child, somehow my daughter and her teachers were able to connect better and move forward. It was like somehow, with all my energy and explosions, I had been keeping

her back ... keeping her shut down. The more anxious I was, the more upset she was. The more settled and comfortable I was in myself, the more open and comfortable she was with others. As I got myself more grounded, she really started making more progress and it was wonderful to see.

Of course, I still had feelings of disappointment or anger – but they were different. They were notched down – they didn't feel like they were going to explode out of my body any minute! The more I learnt to calm my nervous system, the easier it became to see beyond the immediate issues and keep my perspective. I moved into a season of my life – which I'm still enjoying – where there was a *lot* less drama, and a much more settled way of being. And you know – yes, that was good for me, but it was *great* for the rest of my family. I'm actually pretty proud of the journey I took myself on! Learning self-regulation can be such a gift to oneself and others – my only regret is that I didn't realise it sooner.

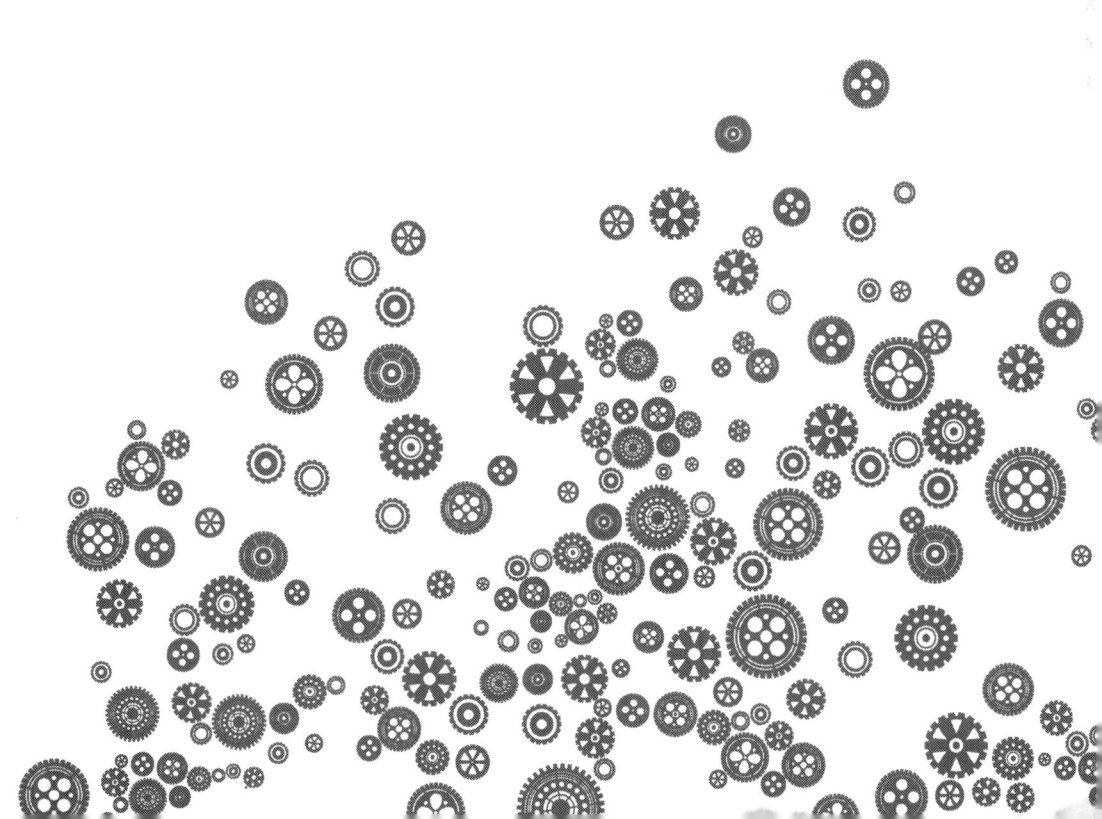

29

Time For Timeout

Children who have had the benefit of watching the adults around them become more proficient at managing themselves – their bodies, their nervous systems – learn. When their key role models acknowledge that getting angry, scared or upset is something that happens to us *all* at times, children pay attention. They relate. They get it. The real learning comes when those same important role models can live out their own commitment to self-regulation around the children.

Children learn that getting angry doesn't have to end in hurting people with hands, feet or words. They learn that feeling scared can be overcome and doesn't have to mean we stop moving forwards, trying things, doing things. Children learn that it is OK to use their voice and they don't need to disappear into freeze when they feel unsafe. As the poem goes, 'children learn what they live'. If we live out a life that is more grounded, they notice. They feel it. They learn it is possible. When they know you have learnt to navigate the path to self-regulation, they get inspired that they can do the same. Children can learn to recognise when their body is getting out of its 'safety' physiology, and they can learn what to do to help themselves when they feel 'unsafe' in anyway.

New skills in PE

Matty's class were all outside. With their teacher away on a course all day, they were being taught by a supply teacher. It was PE.

So what was Matty doing walking purposefully across the playground away from the rest of his class? Why did he have his eyes fixed on the ground in stoic concentration that seemed to be propelling his feet to keep moving at a controlled pace (but not running) all the way to the main school building? He looked as if he was following an invisible line on the concrete, one that he must walk along at all costs. He was on a mission – one that was not yet clear to the Deputy Head, who'd spotted him from the office and stood quietly watching him through the window. Matty had been to the toilet before PE, so that wasn't it. He didn't seem upset, he didn't look unwell, and he was moving in a way not congruent with the laid-back saunter that often beguiled children who'd been sent to 'give someone a message' as a way to get them away from a class (or a teacher) for a few minutes.

Matty came through the door at the same time the Deputy Head 'just happened' to be walking past.

"Alright, Matty?" she asked in her signature way of making a connection, opening the door to communication without directly demanding an answer.

Matty didn't reply. He didn't know what to say. He wasn't sure if he was alright, if things were alright – he was and he wasn't, they were and they weren't.

The Deputy Head changed her question: "I wonder what you are doing in here?"

The non-threatening choice of words, the light tone and sing-song in her voice and sparkle in her eye – all indicating she was almost smiling – reassured Matty that she was just curious: he wasn't in trouble. This helped him. Now he knew what to say, and out it came.

"I came inside because I needed to. He [the supply teacher] is getting stressed out there and so I'm giving him time to calm down. He needs some time out and I came in here to find a safe adult to be with."

That was not what the Deputy Head was expecting to hear. In fact, she realised that, in all her many years' experience as a teacher, she didn't think she had ever experienced this before: a child who is highly sensitive to the energy state of those he is with, recognising that he didn't feel safe when the teacher was getting angry, managing to keep himself grounded enough to keep his neocortex, decision-making brain working, and making a choice to move himself to safety in a controlled manner ...

She didn't know exactly what had gone on outside, but this moment was new to her, and it was certainly new for Matty. His pattern for the past year had been more about a highly reactive nervous system dictating what his body would do in moments like these. He would freeze in the classroom, or get under desks, hide in corners or run out to get himself away. He had fled his classroom regularly, and the whole school building on occasion – never with the awareness, understanding or vocabulary to explain himself.

The work all of them – Matty, his parents, his teachers, in fact the whole school team – had been doing to learn more and more about the role of safety in helping children learn and grow was working. That moment, right there – a moment when the Deputy Head actually felt quietly proud of Matty – was proof. It was a moment of progress for them all.

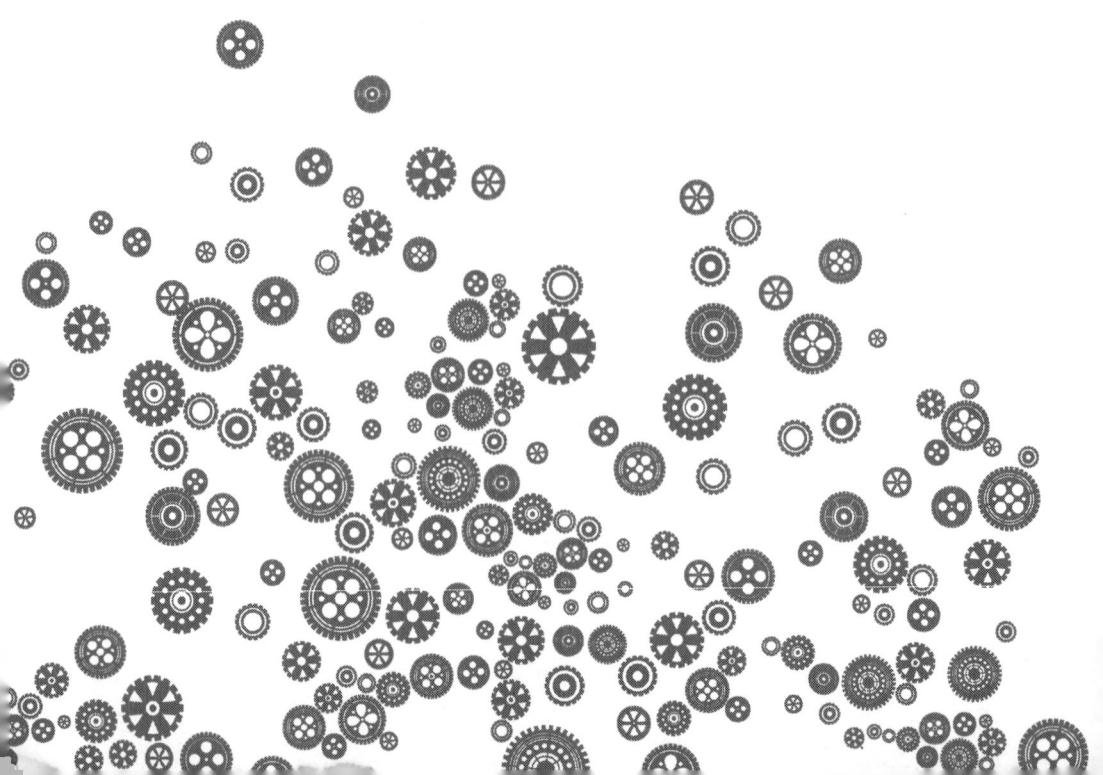

30

From Me To You: A Message To All Who Read This

I nearly didn't write this book.

Most of the people I have come across who are parents, grandparents, teachers or teaching assistants, or who work with children in any other capacity want to do their best by those children. No one wants to be the one to make life harder for children in any way. *We are all doing our best with what we know.*

We all know just how hard it can be to turn up physically and emotionally and care, teach or parent, day in, day out.

When I am working with clients one-to-one, we spend a lot of time noticing and then celebrating the tiny steps. Looking only for the major changes can easily have you feeding disappointment and failure. Disciplining yourself to find the positive in any situation means you will have something solid to use to springboard yourself forwards.

With a mind and heart that wants to cheer and encourage and celebrate any parent or professional who is journeying to understand their children better, I acknowledge that my fear is that you may read this book with an internal voice of self-criticism, turned up high. I know many mums, dads, step-parents, carers and even professionals (who are all humans, too) know that self-critical voice well. The 'it's all my fault, I'm not good enough, I'm to blame' monkey on the shoulder may well take these words I have written and try and beat you down with them.

Please do not let that happen.

Please do not let these words be used to bring you down. That is not my intention.

My hope is that you may find understanding in these words and the stories of the precious people I have shared with you.

I hope that the clarity you get from understanding the things that help your children feel emotionally safe (or not) – which are not all about you, but do include you – will give you power.

I hope that, instead of falling into a guilt pit of "I'm a bad parent/teacher", you will choose the battle cry of wisdom:

"I can see more clearly now – and I use my power to choose where I go from here."

Things can change.

You can change.

Your relationship with your children can change. You can help your children.

You can learn to become more familiar with and responsible for your own body and the messages it gives.

As many times as it takes, you can tread your own path to getting grounded, and you can become a powerful, positive, resource for your tribe.

Remember there are people out there to help you. Seek them out. We all need to hear the voices of those rooting for us, and if you would like to hear me cheering you on personally, then feel free to contact me at claire@groundedgrownups.com.

31

Revisiting Lisa

As we discovered in Chapter 1, Lisa deeply and desperately loved her children, but she couldn't get them to want to talk to her, spend time with her or even be near her.

She had been through numerous traumatic moments and incomprehensible stress over years and her body had got stuck. She had been squeezed by life, and her nervous system was unable to take anymore. She was on full-time high alert and shut-down and, even though she knew the major threat that had chased her life up this mountain into 'freeze' had gone, she couldn't find her way back down. She couldn't find safety. She wasn't grounded. Her girls picked up the subconscious signals and stayed away to protect themselves from her body and its messages. Their neuroception meant they instinctively kept themselves at a distance from her stored anger, her flat face, her internalised terror, her racing heart rate and her muscles racked with tension. She wasn't safe.

What is interesting is that this family, Lisa's family, was restored. It took a bit of time (just a few months), and she did receive help, yet none of the 'usual' or traditional supports were given. She had no parent-coaching, nobody giving her advice on what to do or say to her girls. Neither was there any requirement to talk back through everything that had happened to her.

The help she did receive totally changed her. She learnt how to be friends with her body again; how to notice it and help it; how to follow it, understand it and honour it; and this journey changed the fabric of who she was. It changed the message her body was giving to itself, to the world and to anyone who came near her. Changing the state of her nervous system changed her – her muscles, her breathing, her digestion, her posture, her smile and her grounded-ness. And from that, she became safe.

She was safe to herself and her very body was no longer a threat to her girls. She was safe to come near, and they came. Oh, my word, how they came! The last time I saw Lisa, she told me through smiles and tears of joy how they would now giggle and play-fight with each other over who got to sit nearest to her on the sofa. Her treasures refused to go to bed unless she was there and they had had their goodnight snuggle time with her. The youngest was sleeping better, and Lisa had story after story of different games the older ones asked 'Mummy' to play with them now. She loved working on spelling and reading games with them and she treasured every time they came out of school bursting to let her know when they'd had a wonderful or a bad day. Lisa, the survivor, was so proud of herself. She found the right way to change herself – she became grounded, and that, that changed everything.

References

Amen, D.G. & T. (2016) *The Brain Warrior's Way*. New York: Berkley (Penguin Random House).

Berceli, D. (2008) *The Revolutionary Trauma Release Process: Transcend Your Toughest Times*. Vancouver: Namaste Publishing.

Berceli, D. (2009a) 'Evaluating the effects of stress reduction exercises employing mild tremors: a pilot study'. PhD thesis. University of Arizona. Available at: http://traumaprevention.com/research/ (accessed 17 December 2012).

Berceli, D. (2009b) 'Using the Body to Heal Trauma'. Available at: http://traumaprevention.com/2009/06/27/using-the-body-to-heal-trauma/ (accessed 16 March 2013).

Berceli, D. (2013) 'Tiring Trauma Out: How to Activate the Body's Natural Defense Mechanisms Against Trauma'. Interview by Ruth Buczynski for National Institute for the Clinical Application of Behavioural Medicine. Available at: http://www.nicabm.com/programs/trauma/ (accessed 15 May 2013).

Dykema, R. (2006) 'How your nervous system sabotages your ability to relate': An interview with Stephen Porges about his polyvagal theory. Nexus, March/April, 30–5.

Hill, R. & Castro, E. (2002) *Getting Rid of Ritalin*. Virginia: Hampton Roads Publishing Company Inc.

Kidd, P.M. (2007) 'Omega-3 DHA and EPA for Cognition, Behavior, and Mood: Clinical Findings and Structural-Functional Synergies with Cell Membrane Phospholipids'. *Alternative Medicine Review* 12(3): 207–27. https://pdfs.semanticscholar.org/528b/3d3239146af565ef945fda6bab3746e58722.pdf (accessed 23 May 2016).

Levine, P.A. (2010) *In an Unspoken Voice: How the Body Releases Trauma and Restores Goodness.* Berkeley, CA: North Atlantic Books.

Levine, P.A. & Frederick, A. (1997) *Waking the Tiger: Healing Trauma.* Berkeley, CA: North Atlantic Books.

Oschman, J.L., Chevalier, G. & Brown, R. 'The effects of grounding (earthing) on inflammation, the immune response, wound healing, and prevention and treatment of chronic inflammatory and autoimmune diseases'. *Journal of Inflammation Research* 8 (2015): 83–96. doi:10.2147/JIR.S69656. https://www.ncbi.nlm.nih.gov/pmc/articles/PMC4378297/ (accessed 10 November 2017).

Perry, B. Interview with Guy Macpherson, PhD. Trauma Therapist Podcast Episode 94. https://www.thetraumatherapistproject.com/blog/bruce-perry-md-phd-on-the-trauma-therapist-podcast/ (accessed 6 October 2017).

Porges, S.W. (2004) 'Neuroception: A Subconscious System for Detecting Threats and Safety'. *Zero to Three: Bulletin of the National Center for Clinical Infant Programs* 24(5) (May 2004), 19–24. https://stephenporges.com/images/neuroception.pdf.

Porges, S.W. (2011) *The Polyvagal Theory: Neuropsychological Foundations of Emotions, Attachment, Communication, and Self-Regulation.* (Norton Series on Interpersonal Neurobiology). New York: W.W. Norton & Company.

Porges, S.W. (2017) *The Pocket Guide to the Polyvagal Theory: The Transformative Power of Feeling Safe* (Norton Series on Interpersonal Neurobiology). New York: W.W. Norton & Company.

Porges, S.W. & Buczynski, R. (n.d.), 'The Polyvagal Theory for Treating Trauma'. Transcript of teleseminar session, The National Institute for the Clinical Application of Behavioral Medicine. https://www.nicabm.com (accessed 21 March 2014).

Rothschild, B. (2000) *The Body Remembers: The Psychophysiology of Trauma and Trauma Treatment*. London: W.W. Norton & Company.

Rucklidge, J. (2014) 'The Surprisingly Dramatic Role of Nutrition in Mental Health'. Talk at TEDx Christchurch. https://www.youtube.com/watch?v=3dqXHHCc5lA (accessed 15 December 2014).

Sarris, J. et al. 'Nutritional Medicine as Mainstream in Psychiatry'. *The Lancet Psychiatry* 2(3): 271–4. https://www.thelancet.com/journals/lanpsy/article/PIIS2215-0366(14)00051-0/abstract.

van der Kolk, B. (2014) *The Body Keeps the Score: Brain, Mind and Body in the Healing of Trauma*. New York: Viking.

Wilson, C. (2017) 'A Plea from a Therapist: "Read this before you start counselling"'. http://www.chewinitiatives.com/a-plea-to-anyone-thinking-about-starting-counselling-or-therapy/ (accessed 3 February 2018).

Additional Resources

Websites about TRE

www.traumaprevention.com
If you want to learn more about TRE (Tension Release Exercises) and the research behind it, or to find a registered practitioner anywhere in the world

www.trecollege.com
For more information and a list of active, qualified TRE providers in the UK

> *Remember, if you are interested in exploring TRE, please do so with a trained, qualified and experienced practitioner. It is a wonderful way to work with the body, and works best when the right speed for the individual is established. An experienced practitioner will help you learn how to not go too slow or too fast, and in the way that is just right for your body.*

Other websites

www.seauk.org.uk
Somatic Experiencing Association UK. Learn more about SE or find a practitioner in the UK to work with

www.playtherapy.org
Play Therapy International. For information and a database of qualified Play Therapists internationally

www.bapt.info
British Association of Play Therapists. For information and qualified Play Therapists in the UK

www.playtherapy.org.uk
Play Therapy UK. For information and qualified Play Therapists in the UK

> *Most qualified Play Therapists work with children and/or teens. Some also work with adults*

www.groundedgrownups.com
Online support for parents and professionals wanting to continue this journey of becoming more grounded for themselves and the children they are around

www.chewinitiatives.com
Variety of resources, support and information to help parents and teachers

Books about nervous systems

Reframe your thinking around Autism by Holly Bridges
Further reading on understanding Stephen Porges' Polyvagal Theory and particularly how it applies to autism

The Simple Guide to Child Trauma: What It Is and How to Help by Betsy de Thierry
Further reading for parents and teachers on supporting children who have been through trauma

Trauma is Really Strange by Steve Haines
Further reading for adults to understand trauma and bodies in a comic-book format

What Mental Health Professionals are saying about GROUNDED

"I LOVE this book!
Claire Wilson has taken difficult concepts and made them accessible. I hope this resource is made widely available to everyone who has children in their lives. This will help them to see how they could make small changes which will result in huge changes for the children."
Jan Montgomery, *Accredited Play Therapist, Adult Psychotherapist, trainer*

"As a trauma specialist working with children, I know that the first step towards children being able to heal is for the adults in their life to become grounded as well as knowledgeable. In GROUNDED, Claire Wilson provides an easy-to-understand résumé of how our nervous system works and how adults can use simple techniques to calm themselves. Her use of case study material makes the topic come alive. I enjoyed it immensely and feel it's a very important as well as informative book for parents and those involved with children."
Dr Melanie Salmon, *GP, Gestalt Psychotherapist, TRE trainer and Founder of Quantum Energy Coaching*

"In this insightful and sensitive volume, Claire Wilson provides a powerful narrative that alerts us as adults that '… we cannot write ourselves out of the stories of the children around us.' In Grounded, we learn that teachers, parents, and other adults in the child's world are constantly transmitting their feelings and emotions through subtle bodily cues that may trigger in the child either a sense of danger and uncertainty or a sense of safety and trust.

By integrating constructs from Polyvagal Theory and other neurobiological approaches with personal narratives of the children and adults she has worked with, we experience a greater understanding of how an adult's facial expression, intonation of voice, and general bodily presence can either calm the child or exacerbate aggressive and oppositional behaviors."
Stephen W. Porges, *PhD, Distinguished University Scientist at Indiana University, Professor of Psychiatry at the University of North Carolina, and originator of the Polyvagal Theory.*

- **Do you know more people who might benefit from reading GROUNDED?**

- **Do you have connections with a school or children's charity, however small?**

- **We want to help you get the word out, and do it in a way that helps raise some funds for supporting children too**

I am so aware that charities and even schools are currently struggling to make ends meet, and often a lack of funds leads to vital support services for children being cut.

My goal is to get this book into the hands of as many people who know children as possible.

If you want to *partner with me* to help spread this message around your community, and do so in a way that

    1. allows *your community to buy the book at a significant discount*
    and
    2. brings in *extra funds for your charity or organisation,*

then please get in touch.

Find out more at **www.groundedgrownups.com** or by emailing info@groundedgrownups.com

- **Bulk order options for schools and children's charities from 50 to 500 copies**

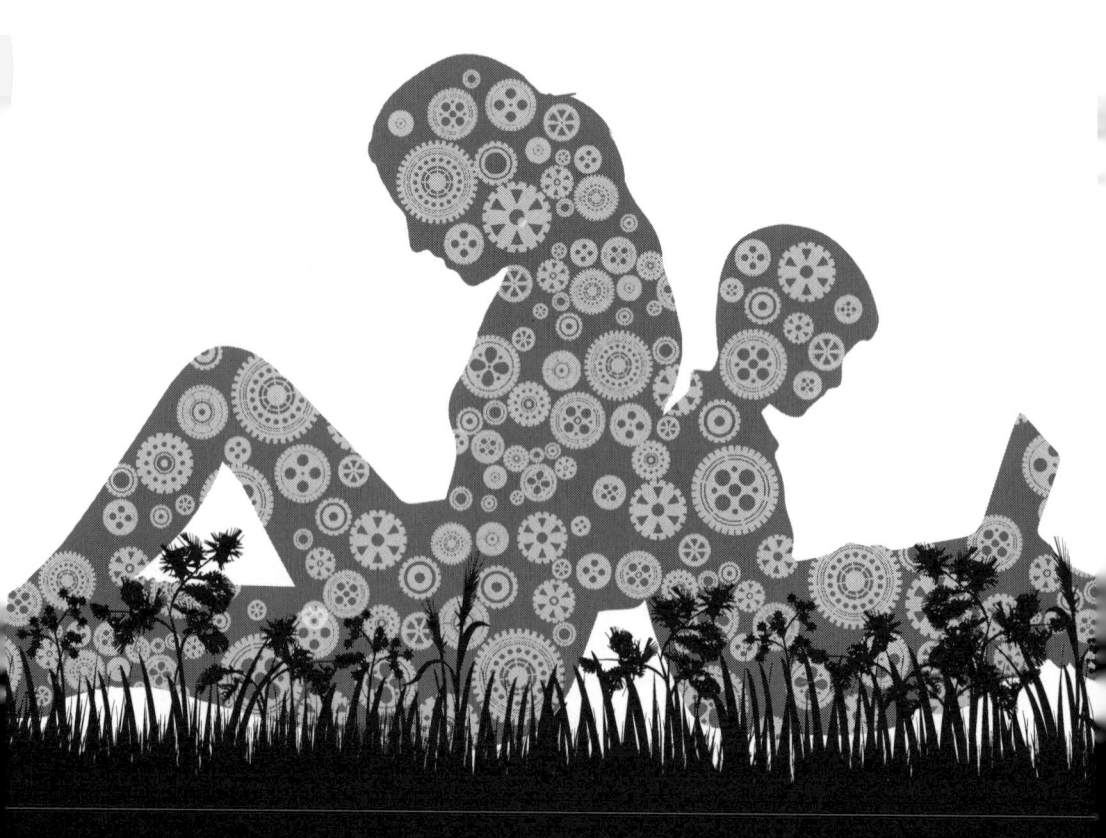

www.groundedgrownups.com